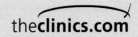
theclinics.com

NEUROIMAGING CLINICS
OF NORTH AMERICA

Pediatric Neurovascular Disease: Diagnosis and Intervention

Guest Editor
PIERRE LASJAUNIAS, MD, PhD

Consulting Editors
MAURICIO CASTILLO, MD, FACR
SURESH K. MUKHERJI, MD

May 2007 • Volume 17 • Number 2

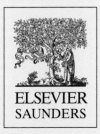

ELSEVIER
SAUNDERS

An imprint of Elsevier, Inc
PHILADELPHIA LONDON TORONTO MONTREAL SYDNEY TOKYO

W.B. SAUNDERS COMPANY

A Division of Elsevier Inc.

1600 John F. Kennedy Boulevard • Suite 1800 • Philadelphia, Pennsylvania 19103-2899

http://www.theclinics.com

NEUROIMAGING CLINICS Volume 17, Number 2
May 2007 ISSN 1052-5149, ISBN-13: 978-1-4160-5321-7, ISBN-10: 1-4160-5321-2

Editor: Lisa Richman

Neuroimaging Clinics (ISSN 1052-5149) is published quarterly by Elsevier Inc., 360 Park Avenue South, New York, NY 10010-1710. Months of issue are February, May, August, and November. Business and editorial offices: 1600 John F. Kennedy Blvd., Suite 1800, Philadelphia, PA 19103-2899. Business and editorial offices: 6277 Sea Harbor Drive, Orlando, FL 32887-4800. Periodicals postage paid at New York, NY, and additional mailing offices. Subscription prices are USD 218 per year for US individuals, USD 336 per year for US institutions, USD 112 per year for US students and residents, USD 252 per year for Canadian individuals, USD 413 per year for Canadian institutions, USD 302 per year for international individuals, USD 413 per year for international institutions and USD 151 per year for Canadian and foreign students and residents. To receive student/resident rate, orders must be accompanied by name of affiliated institution, date of term, and the *signature* of program/residency coordinator on institution letterhead. Orders will be billed at individual rate until proof of status is received. Foreign air speed delivery is included in all *Clinics* subscription prices. All prices are subject to change without notice. POSTMASTER: Send address changes to *Neuroimaging Clinics*, Elsevier Periodicals Customer Service, 6277 Sea Harbor Drive, Orlando, FL 32887-4800. **Customer Service: 1-800-654-2452 (US). From outside of the US, call (+1) 407-345-4000. E-mail: hhspcs@harcourt.com.**

Reprints. For copies of 100 or more, of articles in this publication, please contact the Commercial Reprints Department, Elsevier Inc., 360 Park Avenue South, New York, New York 10010-1710. Tel.: (+1) 212-633-3813; Fax: (+1) 212-462-1935; E-mail: reprints@elsevier.com.

Neuroimaging Clinics is covered by *Excerpta Medica/EMBASE*, the RSNA Index of Imaging Literature, Index Medicus, MEDLINE/MEDLARS, SciSearch, Research Alert, and Neuroscience Citation Index.

Printed in the United States of America.

GOAL STATEMENT

The goal of *Neuroimaging Clinics of North America* is to keep practicing radiologists and radiology residents up to date with current clinical practice in radiology by providing timely articles reviewing the state of the art in patient care.

ACCREDITATION

The *Neuroimaging Clinics of North America* is planned and implemented in accordance with the Essential Areas and Policies of the Accreditation Council for Continuing Medical Education (ACCME) through the joint sponsorship of the University of Virginia School of Medicine and Elsevier. The University of Virginia School of Medicine is accredited by the ACCME to provide continuing medical education for physicians.

The University of Virginia School of Medicine designates this educational activity for a maximum of 60 *AMA PRA Category 1 Credits™*. Physicians should only claim credit commensurate with the extent of their participation in the activity.

The American Medical Association has determined that physicians not licensed in the US who participate in this CME activity are eligible for *AMA PRA Category 1 Credits™*.

Credit can be earned by reading the text material, taking the CME examination online at http://www.theclinics.com/home/cme, and completing the evaluation. After taking the test, you will be required to review any and all incorrect answers. Following completion of the test and evaluation, your credit will be awarded and you may print your certificate.

FACULTY DISCLOSURE/CONFLICT OF INTEREST

The University of Virginia School of Medicine, as an ACCME accredited provider, endorses and strives to comply with the Accreditation Council for Continuing Medical Education (ACCME) Standards of Commercial Support, Commonwealth of Virginia statutes, University of Virginia policies and procedures, and associated federal and private regulations and guidelines on the need for disclosure and monitoring of proprietary and financial interests that may affect the scientific integrity and balance of content delivered in continuing medical education activities under our auspices.

The University of Virginia School of Medicine requires that all CME activities accredited through this institution be developed independently and be scientifically rigorous, balanced and objective in the presentation/discussion of its content, theories and practices.

All authors/editors participating in an accredited CME activity are expected to disclose to the readers relevant financial relationships with commercial entities occurring within the past 12 months (such as grants or research support, employee, consultant, stock holder, member of speakers bureau, etc.). The University of Virginia School of Medicine will employ appropriate mechanisms to resolve potential conflicts of interest to maintain the standards of fair and balanced education to the reader. Questions about specific strategies can be directed to the Office of Continuing Medical Education, University of Virginia School of Medicine, Charlottesville, Virginia.

The authors/editors listed below have identified no professional/financial affiliations for themselves or their spouse/partner:

Ronit Agid, MD; H. Alverez, MD; J.J. Bhattacharya, MD; S. Cullen, MD; Elizabeth A. Eldredge, MD; S. Geibprasert, MD; Tali Jonas-Kimchi, MD; T. Krings, MD, PhD; Pierre Lasjaunias, MD, PhD (Guest Editor); Seon Kyu Lee, MD, PhD; C.B. Luo, MD; R. Garcia-Monaco, MD; Darlene R. Powars, MD; Lisa Richman (Acquisitions Editor); Mark A. Rockoff, MD; G. Rodesch, MD, PhD; M. Sachet, MD; Manohar Shroff, MD; Joon K. Song, MD; Sulpicio G. Soriano, MD; and, Karel G. Ter Brugge, MD.

The authors listed below have identified the following professional/financial affiliations for themselves or their spouse/partner:

Alejandro Berenstein, MD is a consultant for Microvention-Terumo and Siemens Medical System
Yasunari Niimi, MD is a consultant for Terumo Corporation.
A. Ozanne, MD is employed by Bicetre Hospital.
Wing-Yen Wong, MD is employed by Baxter BioScience.

Disclosure of Discussion of non-FDA approved uses for pharmaceutical products and/or medical devices.

The University of Virginia School of Medicine, as an ACCME provider, requires that all authors/editors identify and disclose any "off label" uses for pharmaceutical products and/or for medical devices. The University of Virginia School of Medicine recommends that each reader fully review all the available data on new products or procedures prior to instituting them with patients.

TO ENROLL

To enroll in the Neuroimaging Clinics of North America Continuing Medical Education program, call customer service at 1-800-654-2452 or sign up online at *http://www.theclinics.com/home/cme*. The CME program is available to subscribers for an additional annual fee of USD 175.

PEDIATRIC NEUROVASCULAR DISEASE: DIAGNOSIS AND INTERVENTION

CONSULTING EDITORS

MAURICIO CASTILLO, MD, FACR
Professor and Chief, Section of Neuroradiology, Department of Radiology, University of North Carolina School of Medicine, Chapel Hill, North Carolina

SURESH K. MUKHERJI, MD
Professor and Chief, Neuroradiology and Head and Neck Radiology; Professor, Radiology and Otolaryngology Head and Neck Surgery; and Associate Fellowship Program Director, Department of Radiology, University of Michigan Health System, Ann Arbor, Michigan

GUEST EDITOR

PIERRE LASJAUNIAS, MD, PhD
Service de Neuroradiologie Diagnostique et Thérapeutique, Hôpital Bicêtre, Paris, France

CONTRIBUTORS

RONIT AGID, MD
Assistant Professor, Division of Neuroradiology, Toronto Western Hospital, Department of Medical Imaging, University Health Network (UHN), University of Toronto, Toronto, Ontario, Canada

H. ALVAREZ, MD
Service de Neuroradiologie Diagnostique et Thérapeutique, Hôpital Bicêtre, Paris, France

ALEJANDRO BERENSTEIN, MD
Professor of Radiology, Neurosurgery and Neurology, Hyman-Newman Institute for Neurology and Neurosurgery and the Center for Endovascular Surgery, Roosevelt Hospital, New York, New York; The Albert Einstein College of Medicine

J.J. BHATTACHARYA, MD
Department of Neuroradiology, Institute of Neurological Sciences, Southern General Hospital, Glasgow, UK

S. CULLEN, MD
Department of Radiology and Neurosurgery, Brigham and Women's Hospital, Boston, Massachusetts

ELIZABETH A. ELDREDGE, MD
South Shore Hospital, Weymouth, Massachusetts

S. GEIBPRASERT, MD
Service de Neuroradiologie Diagnostique et Thérapeutique, Hôpital Bicêtre, Paris, France; Department of Radiology, Ramathibodi Hospital Bangkok, Bangkok, Thailand

TALI JONAS KIMCHI, MD
Division of Neuroradiology, Toronto Western Hospital, Department of Medical Imaging, University Health Network (UHN), University of Toronto, Toronto, Ontario, Canada

T. KRINGS, MD, PhD
Service de Neuroradiologie Diagnostique et Thérapeutique, Hôpital Bicêtre, Paris, France; Department of Neuroradiology, University Hospital, University of Technology, Aachen, Germany

PIERRE LASJAUNIAS, MD, PhD
Service de Neuroradiologie Diagnostique et Thérapeutique, Hôpital Bicêtre, Paris, France

SEON KYU LEE, MD, PhD
Assistant Professor, Division of Neuroradiology,
Toronto Western Hospital, Department of Medical
Imaging, University Health Network (UHN),
University of Toronto, Toronto,
Ontario, Canada

C.B. LUO, MD
Department of Radiology, Taipei Veterans General
Hospital, Taipei, Taiwan

R. GARCIA MONACO, MD
Service de Neuroradiologie Diagnostique et
Thérapeutique, Hôpital Bicêtre 78,
Paris, France

YASUNARI NIIMI, MD
Associate Professor of Clinical Radiology and
Neurosurgery, Hyman-Newman Institute for
Neurology and Neurosurgery and the Center for
Endovascular Surgery, Roosevelt Hospital,
New York, New York; The Albert Einstein College
of Medicine

A. OZANNE, MD
Service de Neuroradiologie Thérapeutique, CHU
Bicêtre, Le Kremlin Bicêtre, France

DARLEEN R. POWARS, MD
Department of Pediatrics, Division of
Hematology/Oncology, Women's & Children's
Hospital, Keck School of Medicine at the
University of Southern California, Los Angeles,
California

MARK A. ROCKOFF, MD
Children's Hospital and Harvard Medical School,
Boston, Massachusetts

G. RODESCH, MD, PhD
Service de Neuroradiologie Thérapeutique, CHU
Bicêtre, Le Kremlin Bicêtre, France

M. SACHET, MD
Service de Neuroradiologie Diagnostique et
Thérapeutique, Hôpital Bicêtre 78, Paris, France

MANOHAR SHROFF, MD
Assistant Professor, Division of Neuroradiology,
Department of Radiology, Hospital for Sick
Children, University of Toronto, Toronto, Ontario,
Canada

JOON K. SONG, MD
Hyman-Newman Institute for Neurology
and Neurosurgery and the
Center for Endovascular Surgery, Roosevelt
Hospital, New York, New York; The Albert Einstein
College of Medicine

SULPICIO G. SORIANO, MD
Children's Hospital and Harvard Medical School,
Boston, Massachusetts

KAREL G. TER BRUGGE, MD,
Professor, Division of Neuroradiology, Toronto
Western Hospital, Department of Medical
Imaging, University Health Network (UHN),
University of Toronto, Toronto, Ontario, Canada

WING-YEN WONG, MD
Department of Pediatrics, Division of
Hematology/Oncology, Children's Hospital Los
Angeles, Keck School of Medicine at the University
of Southern California, Los Angeles, California

PEDIATRIC NEUROVASCULAR DISEASE: DIAGNOSIS AND INTERVENTION

Volume 17 • Number 2 • May 2007

Contents

Childhood aneurysms have special characteristics different from adults' aneurysms. Their features were found to significantly differ from aneurysms in adults especially in their gender prevalence, location, morphology and underlying etiology. Treatment options include both surgical and endovascular methods. Whenever possible, endovascular treatment for pediatric aneurysms is the recommended approach, since it offers both reconstructive and deconstructive techniques, durable results and better clinical outcome.

Hemangiomas are vascular tumors that enlarge through proliferation of endothelial cells. They are the most common tumors of infancy, appearing in as many as 10% to 12% of children under 1 year of age, with double this incidence in preterm infants weighing less than 1000 g. Female-to-male predominance is about 4:1. Most hemangiomas appear in the first 6 weeks of life. Hemangiomas can be seen in the skin in 4% to 10% of Caucasian newborns, and less frequently in non-Caucasians. The head and neck regions are involved most frequently, followed by the trunk and the extremities. Despite their benign nature, hemangiomas can cause significant morbidity if not recognized and treated properly. Endovascular treatment is an important component of the interdisciplinary management of hemangiomas.

Arterial Ischemic Stroke in Children

Tali Jonas Kimchi, Ronit Agid, Seon-Kyu Lee, and Karel G. Ter Brugge

Stroke in children is relatively rare. Advances in the clinical recognition and radiographic diagnosis of ischemic stroke have increased the frequency of the diagnosis in infants and children and have raised the need for immediate therapy. A vast amount of data has recently become available through basic research and neuroimaging techniques shedding new light on the chain of events that occur in ischemic stroke in animal models and in the adult population. Whether this new information can also be applied to the pediatric population remains to be seen, but it is likely that the active management of children with acute ischemic stroke in the near future will include brain protection, brain reperfusion, and prevention measures.

Vein of Galen Aneurysmal Malformations

H. Alvarez, R. Garcia Monaco, G. Rodesch, M. Sachet, T. Krings, and Pierre Lasjaunias

Different types of malformations share a dilated vein of Galen, but only one of them is a true vein of Galen aneurysmal malformation (VGAM). The optimal window of opportunity for treatment is between 4 and 5 years of age, because this allows the child to grow and mature. Heart failure and hydrocephalus respond favorably to embolization. Cerebrospinal fluid ventricular shunting, if needed, should be performed after the embolization. The transvenous approach carries significantly elevated morbidity and mortality and is rarely indicated. Anatomic cure of the VGAM is not the main goal of treatment; the ultimate goal is control of the malformation to allow the brain to mature and develop normally.

Diagnosis and Endovascular Treatment of Pediatric Spinal Arteriovenous Shunts

S. Cullen, T. Krings, A. Ozanne, H. Alvarez, G. Rodesch, and Pierre Lasjaunias

Spinal arteriovenous shunts (SAVSs) are rarely diagnosed in infants and children, but they are important clinically because morbidity can be significant. Although these lesions do not form a distinct pathologic group separate from the SAVSs seen in older patients, experience with these malformations in the pediatric population has led to the identification of several important features that are characteristic of this group of SAVSs. Association with genetic abnormalities, heritable (hereditary hemorrhagic telangiectasia) and nonheritable somatic (spinal arteriovenous metameric syndrome or Cobb syndrome), is relatively common and likely underrecognized. Male predominance is more pronounced than in the adult population. Hemorrhagic presentation is more frequent than in adults, except in extremely young children. The natural history seems to be better than previously thought, with early rehemorrhage uncommon. Despite early presentation and severe symptoms, these lesions are frequently amenable to endovascular treatment, often with anatomic cure achieved and with improvement or stabilization of symptoms after partial targeted treatment.

Current Endovascular Management of Maxillofacial Vascular Malformations

Yasunari Niimi, Joon K. Song, and Alejandro Berenstein

Maxillofacial vascular malformations (MFVMs) are formed due to an error of vascular morphogenesis. They generally grow in proportion to the growth of the affected child but may increase in size secondary to various triggering factors such as increased blood flow, arterial occlusion, and venous thrombosis. The development of an individual lesion, especially if it is high flow, may be stimulated by various factors. High flow in an existing MFVM can induce arteriovenous shunting, which, in turn, increases flow demand, cascading enlargement of the malformation. Increased understanding of these additional physiologic variants may help to define their clinical presentation and evolution and assist in designing therapeutic strategies.

Sinovenous thrombosis in children is rare, and the symptoms and signs are nonspecific especially in the neonatal population. MR imaging seems to be the most sensitive for accurate diagnosis of dural sinus thrombosis. General medical and neurologic supportive care is the mainstay of treatment. However, more active medical treatment such as anticoagulation, as well as an aggressive form of treatment such as retrograde transvenous fibrinolytic therapy, in children whose condition declines despite adequate anticoagulation therapy can be justified.

The concept of segmental vascular syndromes with different, seemingly unrelated, diseases is based on the embryology of the neural crest and the mesoderm migration of cells that share the same metameric origin. Migrating patterns of these cells link the brain, the cranial bones, and the face on the same side. A somatic mutation developing in the region of the neural crest or the adjacent cephalic mesoderm before migration can, therefore, be postulated to produce arterial or venous metameric syndromes, including PHACES, CAMS, Cobb syndrome, and Sturge-Weber syndrome. Although these diseases may be rare, their relationships among each other and their postulated linkage with the development of the neural crest and the cephalic mesoderm may shed light on the complex pathology and etiology of various cerebral vascular disorders.

Recent advances in pediatric neurosurgery have drastically improved the outcome in infants and children afflicted with surgical lesions of the central nervous system (CNS). Because most of these techniques were first applied to adults, the physiologic and developmental differences that are inherent in pediatric patients present challenges to neurosurgeons and anesthesiologists alike. The aim of this paper is to highlight these age-dependent approaches to the pediatric neurosurgical patient.

Cerebral vasculopathy in sickle cell anemia (HbSS) is manifest clinically as cerebral infarction and intracranial hemorrhage. The type of stroke, ischemic or hemorrhagic, is age specific with distinct differences in outcomes. Cerebral infarction with or without clinical stroke begins during early childhood and rarely causes death immediately.

ELSEVIER
SAUNDERS

NEUROIMAGING
CLINICS
OF NORTH AMERICA

Neuroimag Clin N Am 17 (2007) xi

Foreword

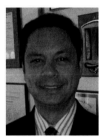 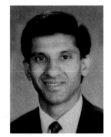

Mauricio Castillo, MD, FACR   Suresh K. Mukherji, MD
Consulting Editors

Mauricio Castillo, MD, FACR
Division of Neuroradiology, Department of Radiology
University of North Carolina School of Medicine
Campus Box 7510, Chapel Hill, NC 27599-7510, USA

E-mail address:
castillo@med.unc.edu (M.Castillo)

Suresh K. Mukherji, MD
Department of Radiology, B2 A209-0030, University of
Michigan Health System, 1500 East Medical Center
Drive, Ann Arbor, MI 48109-0030, USA

E-mail address:
mukherji@umich.edu (S.K. Mukherji)

Interventional neuroradiology continues to expand its applications on almost a daily basis. Just a brief glance at the major neuroradiology and neurosurgery journals shows that a significant percentage of their contents is composed of articles dealing with neurovascular interventions. Not only are radiologists involved; the field now includes other specialties, such as neurosurgeons and neurologists. Most neurointerventional applications are relatively well established and accepted for adult patients. This situation is probably not the case for pediatric patients, in whom their indications are less well established. Moreover, pediatric expertise is less prevalent, mostly because the types of neurologic disorders amenable to minimally invasive forms of treatment are rare in children.

For this issue of *Neuroimaging Clinics of North America*, we are pleased to have a true expert in pediatric neurointervention serve as a guest editor. Pierre Lasjaunias and his team at the Bicêtre Hospital in Paris have pioneered the treatment of many vascular childhood disorders, particularly the vein of Galen malformations. Dr. Lasjaunias has invited to participate in this issue experts from across the world, and the readers of their articles will benefit greatly from the information found in them. One of the benefits of publishing in the Clinics is the fact that the authors are free to express their personal opinions, many of them based on careful clinical observations. Such is the case with many of the articles found in this issue and, in particular, with the article on segmental neurovascular syndromes in children, which we are sure readers will find intriguing. To complement these wonderful articles, we, the consulting editors, have decided to include two related and pertinent articles that have appeared previously in other series of the Clinics. This practice, although not common, is not rare, and we think that it nicely illustrates how different specialties are related. We hope that this issue of *Neuroimaging Clinics* will become a "mini" textbook in the field of pediatric neurointerventional procedures.

doi:10.1016/j.nic.2007.03.009

neuroimaging.theclinics.com

NEUROIMAGING CLINICS OF NORTH AMERICA

Neuroimag Clin N Am 17 (2007) xiii–xiv

Preface

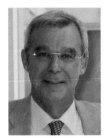

Pierre Lasjaunias, MD, PhD
Hôpital Bicêtre
78 rue du Général Leclerc
Le Kremlin-Bicêtre, France 94275

E-mail address:
pierre.lasjaunias@bct.ap-hop-paris.fr

Pierre Lasjaunias, MD, PhD
Guest Editor

Pediatric neurovascular pathology comprises a group of diverse and rare disorders that are not well known by the medical community. Only rarely can they be approached from traditional nosologic and pathophysiologic angles; unfortunately these classifications are dictated by the technical challenges involved in the care of such patients. For more than 30 years, the staff at the Bicetre Hospital has been involved in the management of pediatric neurovascular diseases. Today, pediatric patients account for about one fourth of all clinical activities and nearly one third of all endovascular procedures at the center. These rare disorders are best treated by highly competent and multidisciplinary medical and technical teams who have gained ample clinical experience with a high number of patients in different age groups. Such experience is difficult to acquire even in large pediatric hospitals and requires long-term follow-up so that therapeutic decisions can be evaluated over the course of time rather than only by satisfactory results immediately after embolization. It was during our association with Alejandro Berenstein and later with Karl ter Brugge that our thoughts on pediatric neurovascular disorders and their relationships to and differences from adult neurovascular disorders matured and became defined. Our goal has been to create rational therapeutic approaches and decision trees that will result in reproducible long-term experiences. Bicetre, New York and Toronto are privileged to serve as training centers for the management of pediatric neurovascular disorders.

Our ongoing wish is to share these experiences and our limitations and doubts in attempting to define therapeutic goals for these rare disorders. Our experience comparing juvenal neurovascular disorders with similar disorders in adults, understanding their anatomy, and describing the techniques and their pitfalls has led to the publication of four books in three volumes, *Surgical Neuroangiography,* of which the first edition took more than 20 years to complete, and the second edition more than 10. The articles in this issue of the *Neuroimaging Clinics of North America* have been written by experts practicing in the three centers previously mentioned. These writings are not exhaustive but are intended to stimulate readers' interest and curiosity. Here, the readers will not find a "cookbook" approach but rather a desire to

doi:10.1016/j.nic.2007.04.001

encourage a professional, ethically and medically responsible approach to dealing with this complex and rare group of disorders. To talk about rare disorders often implies collecting encyclopedic knowledge that sometimes is remote real-world experience. Far away from economical concerns and lucrative research, these rare disorders represent an intellectual challenge and a major public health issue. Despite their rarity, though, the neurovascular diseases in children are contributing largely to the understanding of adult ones, thus, justifying the specific attention being paid to them.

ELSEVIER
SAUNDERS

NEUROIMAGING
CLINICS
OF NORTH AMERICA

Neuroimag Clin N Am 17 (2007) 153–163

Diagnostic Characteristics and Management of Intracranial Aneurysms in Children

Ronit Agid, MD*, Tali Jonas Kimchi, MD, Seon-Kyu Lee, MD, PhD, Karel G. Ter Brugge, MD

Although rare, intracranial aneurysms in children have been discussed thoroughly in the literature [1–13]. Their features have been found to differ significantly from aneurysms in adults, especially in their gender prevalence, location, morphology, and underlying etiology [1,4,14–16]. During the neonatal and infantile period the differences from adult aneurysms are striking, whereas during adolescence the adult aneurysm characteristics become progressively more apparent [17]. The versatility of these aneurysms represents a unique management challenge.

Incidence and gender prevalence

Intracranial aneurysms in the pediatric age group represent less than 5% (0.6%–4.6%) of the total number of intracranial aneurysms in the general population [6]. In children, boys are more likely to harbour aneurysms than are girls [5–8,15,17]. After puberty, this ratio changes to the point that, in adults, women have between three to five times more aneurysms then men [18,19]. In reports that include relatively older children, the male dominance has been less evident [20], with almost a 1:1 ratio between males and females. Others have found a female dominance under the age of 2 years [17].

Clinical presentation

Children with intracranial aneurysms present with subarachnoid hemorrhage about 70% of the time [2,3,9]. The incidence of hemorrhage is reported

Division of Neuroradiology, Toronto Western Hospital, Department of Medical Imaging, University Health Network (UHN), University of Toronto, Toronto, Ontario, Canada
* Corresponding author. Division of Neuroradiology, Toronto Western Hospital, Department of Medical Imaging, 399 Bathurst Street, Toronto, Ontario, M5T 2S8 Canada.
E-mail address: ronit.agid@uhn.on.ca (R. Agid).

doi:10.1016/j.nic.2007.02.001

to be as high as 82% if only infants and children below 5 years of age are considered [21]. Subarachnoid hemorrhage presentation appears to decrease progressively with age and is as low as 45% if only children over 5 years of age are considered [2,8]. Pediatric patients with giant aneurysms present with subarachnoid hemorrhage 35% of the time [22]. Symptoms related to mass effect occur in 20% of all children as the presenting symptom of an intracranial aneurysm [2,21]. Again, this percentage varies among the different age groups and is reported to be as high as 45% in the 5- to 18-year age group [8]. Other clinical presentations such as seizures and stroke are uncommon and occur in less than 10% of cases [2,21].

In the authors' recent series [20], a relatively low percentage of patients presented with subarachnoid hemorrhage when compared with previous series [2,3,9,15]. Children presented most commonly with a neurologic deficit with or without infarct (45%). This presentation was followed by headaches (33%). Subarachnoid hemorrhage or intracerebral hematoma was encountered in 27% of patients. Focal neurologic symptoms including those from mass effect were the most common presentation in some other studies [2,15,17], especially those including older children (5 to 18 years of age) [8], such as in the authors' patient group.

Etiology of aneurysms in children

In children, as in adults, the etiology of aneurysms is mostly unknown. A clear underlying cause for a childhood aneurysm is found in less than 50% of cases [17,20]. Although they are often regarded as congenital [9], as far as being present at birth, neither adult nor pediatric aneurysms are truly congenital in nature [15]. This observation is supported by a large autopsy series that did not detect any incidental aneurysms in children [23]. Thus, the term *congenital aneurysm* to describe aneurysms in children should probably be abandoned, and the identification of an aneurysm in a child should rather raise the suspicion of an underlying disease affecting the blood vessel wall. A review of published histopathology reports of intracranial aneurysms led to the conclusion that a combination of intraluminal, mural, and extravascular factors are likely responsible for the development of saccular aneurysms [24,25]. Lasjaunias and colleagues [15] suggested that aneurysms in children must be the expression of various vessel wall dysfunctions producing transient or permanent failure to repair a partial insult. These included, on one hand, "recognized" mutations and "direct" primary triggers (eg, humoral, immune, infectious, trauma) and, on the other hand, "silent" genetic diseases (eg,

polycystic kidney disease, fibromuscular dysplasia, Ehlers-Danlos syndrome).

There appears to be a clear association between various disease processes that are known to weaken the matrix of the blood vessel wall and the presence of aneurysms in the pediatric age group, and these intramural factors probably have an important role in the etiology of aneurysms in children [26,27]. The concept of "segmental identity and vulnerability" [28] is particularly well illustrated in the aneurysmal vasculopathies in children.

Aneurysms in children are traditionally referred to according to their underlying etiology (eg, traumatic, infectious). Because a clear underlying cause for a childhood aneurysm is found in less then 50% of cases [17,20], with the lack of a known underlying condition, the remaining aneurysms are named according to their appearance on angiography. Aneurysms are called "berry" or "saccular" when they have a saccular appearance and "dissecting" when the aneurysm has a fusiform appearance and has pre- or postaneurysmal narrowing [20]. The incidence of each type of aneurysm must be adjusted to the patient's age at presentation. Dissections are dominant during the first 5 years of life, whereas saccular aneurysms are more common in children older than 6 years.

Traumatic aneurysms

Traumatic aneurysms account for about 5% to 39% of pediatric aneurysms [2,15,17,20,21,29,30]. Of these, about 40% involve the distal anterior cerebral artery complex (adjacent to the falx), 35% involve the major vessels along the skull base, and 25% are cortical in location [29–31]. These children usually present with a hemorrhagic episode 3 to 4 weeks after injury, but immediate bleeding has also been reported [32]. Seventy two percent of children have sustained a closed head injury, 16% a penetrating injury, and the remainder a history of various types of injuries, including surgery [30,32,33]. Most post-traumatic aneurysms increase in size on angiographic follow-up before treatment [31]. This finding is secondary to a false or pseudoaneurysm that corresponds to an extravascular space, usually within a hematoma surrounding the aneurysm. Although the evolution of these lesions can sometimes be favorable with spontaneous healing of the leakage point, a mortality rate of 31% has been reported [34].

Infectious aneurysms

Infectious aneurysms account for 5% to 15% of pediatric aneurysms [1,2,10,21]. The term *mycotic arterial aneurysm* was proposed by Osler in 1901 to describe aneurysms seen during bacterial endo-carditis. This designation has been kept to identify aneurysms associated with an infectious state [35]. Today, the term *infectious arterial aneurysm* seems more appropriate [36]. Infectious arterial aneurysms may involve the artery directly by continuity from sphenoid sinus or mastoid air cell infections with osteomyelitis and sinus thrombophlebitis or reach the artery via infectious emboli [20,37,38]. A direct involvement of the arterial wall is the mechanism most often advocated, with an infectious process progressing from the lumen to the extravascular space [39,40]. Although these aneurysms can be caused by fungal infections, they are most often of bacterial origin [39,41,42]. The most common organism is staphylococcus, followed by streptococcus and other gram-negative organisms [21]. Infectious arterial aneurysms often complicate bacterial endocarditis in infants with congenital or rheumatic heart disease. The time interval between the infectious embolus and the development of an infectious arterial aneurysm including rupture can be as short as 24 to 48 hours. Twenty percent of children with aneurysms of infectious origin die despite antibiotic treatment (**Fig. 1**) [20,21].

Infectious arterial aneurysms associated with HIV

Several reports of aneurysms in children associated with HIV are found in the literature [17,43–46]. In children, neurovascular manifestations of AIDS differ markedly from those in adults. Whereas vascular complications in adults usually consist of vascular occlusions associated with distal emboli and complications of thrombocytopenia, in children, cerebrovascular lesions are mostly due to arteritis including arterial sclerosis, vascular occlusions, and the formation of intracranial aneurysms [45,47,48]. A few cases of HIV-infected children with multiple fusiform aneurysms have been described [46]. These aneurysms were almost all multifocal fusiform arterial dilatations involving the major vessels of the circle of Willis, predominantly involving the supraclinoid internal carotid artery as well as the basilar artery, not affecting the distal parts of the cerebral arteries. The distal arterial segments showed mostly a typical appearance of arteritis including stenosis and thrombosis [46].

The pathogenesis of fusiform aneurysms in HIV-infected children has been discussed by several investigators [45,47,49] and remains controversial. Some have proposed the vasculopathy to be secondary to an infectious cause [47,49]. However, it seems that primary arterial wall infection is unlikely, because histologic and bacteriologic analyses of these lesions failed to detect the presence of any infectious agent, and none of the patients had

a laboratory confirmed central nervous system infection at the time of the diagnosis. Shah and colleagues [48] suggested that the aneurysms (as well as the arterial thromboses and stenoses) seen in this population with severe immune deficiencies were in fact inflammatory panarteritic lesions involving the vasa vasorum and adventitia, causing ischemia of the arterial wall leading to the destruction of the lamina elastica.

Although childhood HIV lesions were initially considered as relatively specific [49], similar features have been observed in chronic mucocutaneous candidiasis (CMCC) [50]. CMCC is a rare familial primary immunodeficiency of unknown etiology characterized by recurrent infections of the mucous membranes, nails, and skin with *Candida albicans* [46,50,51]. The association of CMCC with cerebral vasculitis or aneurysm is rare, but the similarities between cerebral aneurysms in CMCC and AIDS are remarkable. CMCC aneurysms are fusiform and present in the same topographic distribution involving the vessels of the base and sparing of the distal territories. This observation supports the concept of "segmental susceptibility" of the cerebral arterial system [28]. It is possible that intracranial aneurysms occurring in children who have CMCC or AIDS reveal areas of the cerebral vasculature that apparently share the same "identity" or vulnerability [52]. The immune disease exposes these areas to specific or nonspecific triggers depending on the pre-existence of a segmental structural weakness.

Aneurysms associated with vascular conditions

A variety of case reports have described the association of aneurysms in the pediatric population with systemic disorders such as collagen vascular diseases. Ehlers-Danlos syndrome, Klippel-Trenaunay syndrome, hereditary hemorrhagic telangiectasia, tuberous sclerosis, moyamoya syndrome, coarctation of the aorta, and fibromuscular hyperplasia have all been documented to occur in association with aneurysms in children [26,27,53,54]. These disease processes that are known to weaken the matrix of the blood vessel wall are clearly associated with the presence of aneurysms in the pediatric age group.

Saccular aneurysms

Most of the aneurysms in the pediatric population (between 46% and 70%) are reported to be of this type [2,17,20,21]. The etiology of saccular aneurysms remains as controversial in the pediatric age group as in adults. Despite their location at the

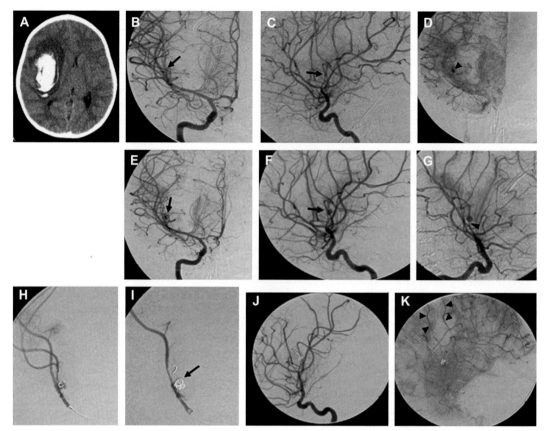

Fig. 1. Infectious aneurysm. Five-year-old girl presenting with left sided hemiparesis 2 weeks post viral infection. The patient did not improve clinically on antibiotic treatment and a lumbar puncture showed elevated white blood cell count and red blood cells. (*A*) Non enhanced CT revealed a large intra-parenchymal hemorrhage. (*B–D*) Cerebral angiogram at presentation (in AP (*B+D*) and lateral (*C*) views) demonstrated a fusiform aneurysm on one of the M2 branches of the right MCA (*arrow*) with stagnation of contrast within the aneurismal sac (*arrow head* in *D*). (*E–G*) A cerebral angiogram performed three days later (in AP (*E*), lateral (*F*) and oblique (*G*) views) show significant aneurismal growth; in addition pre-aneurysmal stenosis is clearly appreciated on the oblique view (*arrow head* in *G*). (*H–I*) AP views of a selective angiogram through a microcathter positioned in the parent vessel shows the coiling of the aneurysm, with partial obliteration (*H*) followed by complete obliteration of aneurysm and sacrifice of the parent M2 branch (*I*). (*J–K*) Post treatment lateral angiogram of the left ICA (arterial phase (*J*) and late parenchymal blush phase (*K*)) demonstrates lack of opacification and of parenchymal blush of the arterial territory previously supplied by the sacrificed vessel. Retrograde flow via leptomeningeal collaterals into the occluded vessels is noted on the later phase (*arrow heads* in *K*).

bifurcation point of various vessels, intrinsic hemodynamic factors almost certainly have less of a role in children as compared with in adults. Mural or systemic factors are considered to be more important [15].

Dissecting aneurysms (nontraumatic)

The frequency of dissecting aneurysms in the pediatric age group is four times that in adults [17,20]. This type of aneurysm tends to be located at the posterior circulation, especially the P1 and P2 segments of the posterior cerebral artery, supraclinoid internal carotid artery, and middle cerebral artery [20,24]. In the authors' experience, most dissecting

aneurysms have involved the posterior circulation [20], which was also true in more than 50% of Lasjaunias' recent series [17]. Both of these recent series contained a larger number of nontraumatic dissecting aneurysms (18.9% in the authors' series, 45% in Lasjaunias' series) when compared with the numbers reported previously in the literature [55–57].

The focal arterial stenotic segments that are often observed proximal or distal to a dissecting aneurysm suggest mural damage. Stenotic vessel wall can induce spontaneous thrombosis, and some of the dissecting aneurysms in children heal spontaneously, leading to occlusion of the parent artery [58]. This occlusion is often well tolerated in the child owing to good collateral circulation via the circle of Willis or pial collateral anastomoses. In the Lasjaunias' series, the time frame for spontaneous thrombosis of dissecting aneurysms was 3 weeks to 7 months [17].

Two types of dissections can be encountered [17,20]. The first type involves extensive vessel wall damage (fusiform or wide neck "saccular" aneurysms) without evidence of mural hematoma. These aneurysms may present with a deep-seated stroke or a subarachnoid hemorrhage. Early recurrence of rupture often occurs during the first few days, and aggressive treatment is recommended. In the second type, focal lesions can be of large size (giant or large "saccular" aneurysms) with evidence of recent mural hematoma on CT or MR imaging but with no subarachnoid hemorrhage. Presentation is often ischemic, and spontaneous healing with completion of the lumen thrombosis is frequently observed. Medical treatment with aspirin or even anticoagulation is recommended;

anti-inflammatory treatment may have to be discussed (Fig. 2) [59].

Giant aneurysms

Giant aneurysms are known to be of increased incidence in children, being about four times more common than in adults [15]. Their reported incidence in this age group is between 20% and 45% [2,5,8,20–22]. Giant aneurysms should not only be distinguished because of their size but also as a group within the dissection category. Repeated small intramural hematomas may lead to formation of the onionskin pattern of thrombotic layers on CT and MR imaging. Children who have giant size aneurysms often present with mass effect and only 35% of the time with subarachnoid hemorrhage [20,22]. The natural history of these unruptured aneurysms varies depending on their size (Fig. 3) [18].

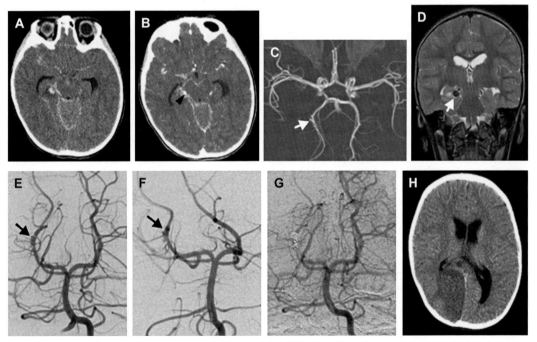

Fig. 2. Non-traumatic dissecting aneurysm. A 5 year old girl that was found unresponsive and later developed sixth nerve palsy and double vision. (*A*) Unenhanced axial CT at presentation shows Fisher grade I subarachnoid hemorrhage (SAH). (*B*) Contrast enhanced axial CT reveals a round enhancing "pocket" of contrast within the right ambient cistern (*arrowhead*). (*C–D*) MRI: Coronal T2 weighted MRI image (*D*) demonstrates a round area of flow void (*arrow*), corresponding to aneurysmal dilatation (*arrow*) of the right posterior cerebral artery (PCA) as seen on MR angiogram (*C*). (*E–F*) Intra-arterial cerebral angiogram of the left vertebral artery in towns (*E*) and oblique (*F*) views demonstrate a fusiform aneurysm of the P2-3 segment of the right PCA with pre and post aneurismal stenoses suggesting dissection (*arrow*). (*G*) Towns view of the left vertebral artery after endovascular coiling of the aneurysm and sacrifice of parent vessel. (*H*) Non-enhanced axial CT 5 days post treatment reveals an infarct in right PCA territory. The patient made a good clinical recovery but suffers from homonimus hemianopsia.

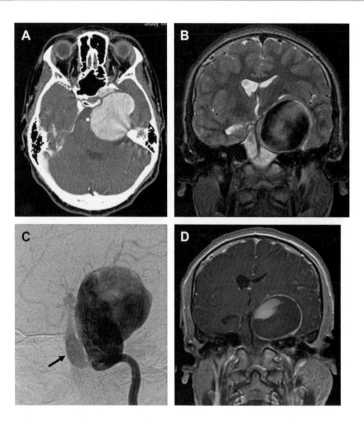

Fig. 3. Giant aneurysm. Twelve-year-old boy presenting with double vision due to left sided 6th nerve palsy. (*A*) Axial contrast enhanced CT angiogram demonstrates a large (5.5 cm in diameter) enhancing aneurysm compressing the pons and the left temporal lobe (*B*). (*B*) Coronal T2 weighted image shows the giant aneurysm as a large flow void displacing the basilar artery. (*C*) Cerebral angiogram of the left internal carotid artery (ICA) in lateral view reveals a fusiform aneurysm arising from the petrous segment of the ICA with a dysplastic arterial segment distal to the aneurysm (*arrow*). (*D*) Contrast enhanced coronal T1 weighted image 3 days after surgical treatment with trapping of the aneurysm and sacrifice of the parent ICA demonstrates a thrombosed aneurysm with enhancement of the aneurismal wall.

Location of childhood aneurysms

The bifurcation of the internal carotid artery is the most common single site for aneurysms in children [3,6,10–12,15,20]. In fact, children have a fivefold increased incidence of carotid artery termination aneurysms, with an incidence of 24% to 54% for this location [6,8,10–12] compared with an incidence of less than 5% in adults [19]. The anterior communicating artery, which is the single most common location for aneurysms in adults [19], is rarely involved in infants and young children but becomes the most common site (35%) in children aged more than 15 years [10].

Children have a much higher incidence of posterior circulation aneurysms when compared with adults [5,7,9,11,20], reaching 29.7% in Toronto's recent series [20]. This is probably due to the fact that dissecting aneurysms that are prevalent in children are commonly situated posteriorly [20,60].

In the two large series reported recently [17,20], an interesting observation was made linking location to etiology. Although the most common location of infectious traumatic and saccular aneurysms was the carotid termination followed by the anterior communicating artery, dissecting aneurysms were more commonly located in the posterior

circulation followed by the intradural portion of the internal carotid artery (Fig. 4) [17,20].

Multiplicity of aneurysms in children

The incidence of multiple aneurysms in the same patient in children has been reported to be considerably lower than that in adults [1,13,15,19–21]. The likelihood of multiplicity of lesions in a given child depends on the etiology of the aneurysm [17,20,46]. In a review by Choux and colleagues [21], only 2% of children with saccular aneurysms showed multiplicity, whereas it was more common (15%) in children with aneurysms of infectious origin. In fact, the multiplicity of saccular aneurysms in children is low in comparison with that in adults but is high when the dissecting aneurysms are considered and even more so among the infectious and immune compromised patients. This observation is supported by the authors' recent study in which two of three patients with multiple aneurysms had an underlying infection or immune etiology, and only one patient had multiple berry aneurysms [20].

Familial occurrence

Familial occurrence has been reported in children [61–63] but appears to be less frequent than in

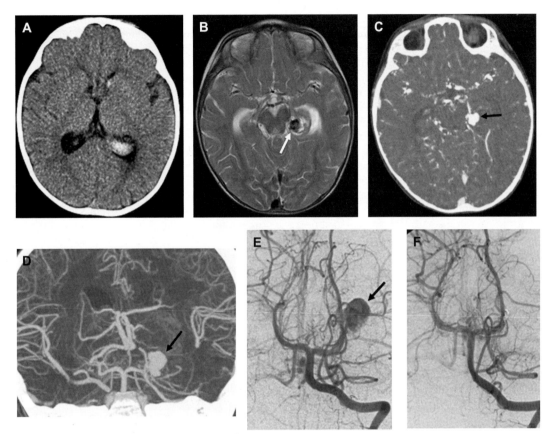

Fig. 4. Dissecting aneurysm. Therteen months old girl, admitted due to drowsiness and vomiting. (*A*) Non-enhanced axial CT revealed intra-ventricular SAH. (*B*) Axial T2 weighted MRI shows a round flow void in the left ambient cistern (*arrow*). (*C–D*) Contrast enhanced CT angiogram: axial cut (*C*) and coronal MIP reconstruction (*D*) demonstrated a 1 cm in diameter aneurysm (*arrow*) off the left PCA at P2-3 segment. (*E–F*) Towns view of intra-arterial angiogram of the left vertebral artery. (*E*) Prior to treatment (*arrow points* to aneurysm) and (*F*) after coil obliteration of the aneurysm and sacrifice of parent vessel. The patient made an excellent clinical recovery with no infarct.

adults. This observation might reflect either the restricted application of neuroimaging in the pediatric population or the role played by unknown triggers over time that is needed to morphologically reveal an aneurysm. The association of autosomal dominant polycystic kidney disease and intracranial aneurysms is well known in adults but is rare in children. The association of the recessive form of polycystic kidney disease and aneurysms is exceptional [64].

Treatment strategies and outcome

The currently available treatment options for pediatric aneurysms include open surgery, an endovascular approach, and conservative management. Conservative management is reserved for some of the dissecting aneurysms that can be treated with anticoagulation or for specific cases of infectious aneurysms that are treated with antibiotics. Conservative supportive management is sometimes chosen when no good treatment option is available and for children in grave clinical condition.

Open surgery and the endovascular approach both offer reconstructive and deconstructive options, that is, excluding the aneurysm from the blood stream while preserving the parent vessel versus occlusion of the aneurysm together with its parent vessel. Both open surgery and endovascular treatment are appropriate for saccular, fusiform, and giant aneurysms. The main issue when proceeding from open surgery to endovascular treatment is the fact that surgery has a good outcome in 60% to 80% of children presenting with saccular aneurysms [1,10], with a reported mortality rate of 20% that reflects the natural history of the disease and the surgical difficulty [4,21].

Balloon occlusion of large aneurysms with sacrifice of the parent vessel was first reported in a child by Lapresle and colleagues [65] and subsequently by Higashida and colleagues [66] and Banna and colleagues [67] with a good outcome. Numaguchi and colleagues [68] described a successful case of intra-aneurysmal deposition of platinum coils in a child. Endovascular treatment for pediatric aneurysms is following the path of endovascular treatment of vascular malformations in children and of aneurysms in adults [4,19,66]. When treating aneurysms, the goal should be not only to achieve alleviation of the acute symptoms (eg, owing to mass effect) but also to protect the patient from a future bleed. An endovascular approach can only be considered if it achieves both goals.

Most of the literature on the results of endovascular treatment for pediatric aneurysms comprises case reports [54,69–71], with only a few publications reporting the outcome of larger series [3,14,15,17,20,72]. Most of the case reports present a good outcome and successful occlusion of the aneurysm with reconstructive or deconstructive methods [17,20,27,54,68–70]. Rarely, a good immediate outcome but with late re-bleeding and death [69] or simply treatable recurrence of aneurysm [72] has been reported. Over the last 15 years, there has been a gradual shift from traditional surgical approaches toward endovascular treatment of aneurysms. This trend is increasing as interventional skills grow, new tools and techniques are developed, and experience with adult aneurysms shows superior results for endovascular treatment [18,19]. An evaluation of the combined experience of the Hopital de Bicetre, Paris, and the Toronto Western Hospital including nearly 100 cases showed the following overall management: 20% of the aneurysms were treated surgically, 50% were treated by endovascular means, and 30% were managed conservatively [17,20]. These recently published series conclude that, as is true in adults, the endovascular approach should be preferred in children whenever technically possible [17,20]. In the Toronto experience, patients treated by endovascular means had a better clinical outcome than children treated by surgery [20]. Although one group has recently raised concern regarding the long-term results of endovascular treatment in the pediatric population [72], the authors' experience with relatively long-term follow-up shows no re-bleeds after endovascular treatment and strongly supports favoring endovascular treatment for pediatric aneurysms [17,20].

Treatment for specific types of aneurysms

Traumatic aneurysms can be treated surgically or endovascularly mainly by deconstructive techniques such as occlusion of the aneurysm and parent vessel sacrifice [17,20,32]. Differentiating false from dissecting aneurysms is crucial. Endovascular filling of a ruptured false pouch should be avoided or at least performed under very restrictive conditions [17].

Infectious aneurysms are primarily treated with antibiotics, but, in some instances, early clipping or coiling has been performed [17,20,38]. Early endovascular management is sometimes mandatory for infectious aneurysms responding poorly or not at all to conservative treatment [36,38]. This management may require sacrifice of the involved arterial segment because these aneurysms are commonly fusiform. The need to treat several locations or unruptured infectious aneurysms warrants discussion for each specific case, taking into consideration the response of the underlying infectious process to antibiotics, the morphologic changes of the aneurysm under appropriate treatment, and the postulated risk carried by certain locations in case of hemorrhage. The need for anticoagulation in some specific cardiac situations may also prompt intervention. Surgery has little to add in this pathology unless a decompressive operation for intracranial hemorrhage needs to be performed.

Nontraumatic dissecting aneurysms are difficult to manage because they may form on a dysplastic artery and tend to be unstable and re-bleed rapidly [17]. They often require endovascular parent artery occlusion as treatment [17,20]. Dissecting aneurysms of the middle cerebral artery (M1 segment) or anterior cerebral artery (A1 segment) are the most difficult cases to manage because of the involvement of perforating arteries arising from the dissected aneurysmal wall. Parent artery sacrifice is often not done early enough in view of its eloquence and the feared risk for associated neurologic deficit. In these instances, surgery faces the same challenge with a paper-thin arterial wall. Dissecting aneurysms presenting with deep-seated ischemic infarcts should be analyzed with great care.

For giant aneurysms, surgical treatment mostly consists of trapping, proximal occlusion, and various bypass procedures, and, in less than 30%, surgical clipping of the aneurysm [73]. An endovascular approach offers both trapping and proximal occlusion. If a bypass is needed, surgery is the more natural choice, although a combined approach is also an option [3]. Antiplatelet medication such as aspirin as a preventive measure can be used to prevent distal stroke of thrombotic origin from a large partially thrombosed aneurysm or following the sacrifice of the parent vessel in a giant aneurysm [17].

Clinical outcome

In the recent Toronto series [20], children treated by endovascular means had a better clinical outcome than in the surgically treated group. Seventy seven percent of the patients who received endovascular treatment made a good recovery (modified Rankin scale of 0–1) compared with 44.4% of the patients treated by open surgery. Only 23% of patients treated endovascularly were left with a significant neurologic deficit (modified Rankin scale of 2–5) versus 44.4% of the patients treated by open surgery. This observation was made despite no significant difference in the clinical grade (Hunt and Hess) at presentation in the two groups. No rebleeds were encountered in endovascularly treated or surgically treated patients. This study had a relatively long follow-up period (2 months to 12 years), which is especially important in children. Lasjaunias and colleagues [17] also reported good long-term results and outcome in their endovascularly treated pediatric aneurysms.

Regarding conservatively treated patients, most of these patients make a good recovery, whereas the prognosis for the rest is grave [15,17,20]. This observation is most likely secondary to the fact that patients included in this group are divided into those who are very ill clinically and those who have a relatively good prognosis requiring only supportive medical care.

Summary

Childhood aneurysms have special characteristics different from aneurysms in adults. This fact warrants a detailed search for the disease process that leads to their development because it will enable prevention, screening, and, most importantly, a mechanism-derived treatment approach. In the mean time, whenever possible, endovascular treatment for pediatric aneurysms is the recommended approach because it offers both reconstructive and deconstructive techniques, durable results, and a better clinical outcome when compared with surgery.

References

[1] Kanaan I, Lesjaunias P, Coats R. The spectrum of intracranial aneurysms in pediatrics. Minim Invasive Neurosurg 1995;38:1–9.

[2] Herman JM, Rekate HL, Spetzler RF. Pediatric intracranial aneurysms: simple and complex cases. Pediatr Neurosurg 1991–1992;17:66–73

[3] Proust F, Toussaint P, Garnieri J, et al. Pediatric cerebral aneurysms. J Neurosurg 2001;94:733–9.

[4] Lasjaunias P, Terbrugge KG, Berenstein A. Intracranial aneurysms in children. In: Surgical neuroangiography 3: clinical and interventional aspects in children. Berlin: Springer-Verlag; 2006. p. 789–836.

[5] Meyer FB, Sundt TM Jr, Fode NC, et al. Cerebral aneurysms in childhood and adolescence. J Neurosurg 1989;70:420–5.

[6] Patel AN, Richardson AE. Ruptured intracranial aneurysms in the first two decades of life: a study of 58 patients. J Neurosurg 1971;35:571–6.

[7] Amacher LA, Drake CG. Cerebral artery aneurysms in infancy, childhood and adolescence. Childs Brain 1975;1:72–80.

[8] Gerosa M, Licata C, Fiore DL, et al. Intracranial aneurysms of childhood. Childs Brain 1980;6: 295–302.

[9] Allison JW, Davis PC, Sato Y, et al. Intracranial aneurysms in infants and children. Pediatr Radiol 1998;28:223–9.

[10] Pasqualin A, Mazza C, Cavazzani P, et al. Intracranial aneurysms and subarachnoid hemorrhage in children and adolescents. Childs Nerv Syst 1986;2:185–90.

[11] Storrs BB, Humphreys RP, Hendrick EB, et al. Intracranial aneurysms in the pediatric age-group. Childs Brain 1982;9:358–61.

[12] Almeida GM, Pindaro J, Plese P, et al. Intracranial arterial aneurysms in infancy and childhood. Childs Brain 1977;3:193–9.

[13] Ostergaard JR, Voldby B. Intracranial arterial aneurysms in children and adolescents. J Neurosurg 1983;58:832–7.

[14] Laughlin S, Terbrugge KG, Willinsky RA, et al. Endovascular management of pediatric intracranial aneurysms. Interventional Neuroradiology 1997;3(3):205–14.

[15] Lasjaunias PL, Campi A, Rodesch G, et al. Aneurysmal disease in children: review of 20 cases with intracranial arterial localisations. Interventional Neuroradiology 1997;3:215–29.

[16] terBrugge KG. Neurointerventional procedures in the pediatric age group. Childs Nerv Syst 1999;15:751–4.

[17] Lasjaunias P, Wuppalapati S, Alvarez H, et al. Intracranial aneurysms in children aged under 15 years: review of 59 consecutive children with 75 aneurysms. Childs Nerv Syst 2005;21(6): 437–50.

[18] International Study of Unruptured Intracranial Aneurysms Investigators. Unruptured intracranial aneurysms: natural history, clinical outcome, and risks of surgical and endovascular treatment. Lancet 2003;362:103–10.

[19] International Subarachnoid Aneurysm Trial (ISAT) Collaborative Group. International subarachnoid aneurysm trial (ISAT) of neurosurgical clipping versus endovascular coiling in 2143 patients with ruptured intracranial aneurysms: a randomized trial. Lancet 2002;360: 1267–74.

[20] Agid R, Souza MP, Reintamm G, et al. The role of endovascular treatment for pediatric aneurysms. Childs Nerv Syst 2005;21(12):1030–6.

[21] Choux M, Lena G, Genitori L. Intracranial aneurysms in children. In: Raimondi A, Choux M, Di Rocco C, editors. Cerebrovascular

disease in children. Vienna (Austria): Springer; 1992. p. 123–31.

[22] Peerless SJ, Nemoto S, Drake CG. Giant intracranial aneurysms in children and adolescents. In: Edwards MSB, Hoffman HJ, editors. Cerebral vascular disease in children and adolescents. Baltimore (MD): William and Wilkins; 1989.

[23] Housepian EM, Pool JA. A systemic analysis of intracranial aneurysms from the autopsy file of the Presbyterian Hospital, 1914 to 1956. J Neuropathol Exp Neurol 1958;17:409–23.

[24] Stehbens WE. Histopathology of cerebral aneurysms. Arch Neurol 1958;17:409–23.

[25] Stehbens WE. Ultrastructure of aneurysms. Arch Neurol 1975;32:798–807.

[26] Pope FM, Kendall BE, Slapak GI, et al. Type III collagen mutations causes fragile cerebral arteries. Br J Neurosurg 1991;5:551–74.

[27] Taira T, Tamura Y, Kawamura H. Intracranial aneurysm in a child with Klippel-Trenaunay-Weber syndrome: case report. Surg Neurol 1991;36: 303–6.

[28] Lasjaunias P. Segmental identity and vulnerability in cerebral arteries. Interventional Neuroradiology 2000;6:113–24.

[29] Yazbak PA, McComb JG, Raffel C. Pediatric traumatic intracranial aneurysms. Pediatr Neurosurg 1955;22:15–9.

[30] Ventureyra EC, Higgins MJ. Traumatic intracranial aneurysms in childhood and adolescence: case reports and review of the literature. Childs Nerv Syst 1994;10:361–79.

[31] Nakstad P, Nornes H, Hauge HN. Traumatic aneurysms of the pericallosal arteries. Neuroradiology 1986;28:335–8.

[32] Kneyber MC, Rinkel GJ, Ramos LM, et al. Early posttraumatic subarachnoid hemorrhage due to dissecting aneurysms in three children. Neurology 2005;65(10):1663–5.

[33] Sutton LN. Vascular complications of surgery for craniopharyngioma and hypothalamic glioma. Pediatr Neurosurg 1994;21:124–8.

[34] Buckingham MJ, Crone KR, Ball WS, et al. Traumatic intracranial aneurysms in childhood: two cases and a review of the literature. Neurosurgery 1988;22(2):398–408.

[35] Hurst RW, Kagetsu NJ, Berenstein A. Angiographic findings in two cases of aneurysmal malformation of vein of Galen prior to spontaneous thrombosis: therapeutic implication. AJNR Am J Neuroradiol 1992;13:1446–50.

[36] Micheli F, Schteinschnaider A, Plaghos LL, et al. Bacterial cavernous sinus aneurysm treated by detachable balloon technique. Stroke 1989; 20(12):1751–4.

[37] Suwanwela C, Suwanwela N, Charuchinda S, et al. Intracranial mycotic aneurysms of extravascular origin. J Neurosurg 1972;36(5):552–9.

[38] Marsot-Dupuch K, Riachi S, Berthet K, et al. Infectious aneurysms of the cavernous carotid artery. J Radiol 2000;81(8):891–8.

[39] Barrow DL, Prats AR. Infectious intracranial aneurysm: comparison of groups with and without endocarditis. Neurosurgery 1990;27:562–73.

[40] Clare CE, Barrow DL. Infectious intracranial aneurysms. Neurosurg Clin N Am 1992;3:551–66.

[41] Bohmfalk GL, Story JL, Wissinger JP, et al. Bacterial intracranial aneurysm. J Neurosurg 1978; 48(3):369–82.

[42] Horten BC, Abbott GF, Porro RS. Fungal aneurysms of intracranial vessels. Arch Neurol 1976; 8:577–9.

[43] Husson RN, Saini R, Lewis LL, et al. Cerebral artery aneurysms in children infected with human immunodeficiency virus. J Neurosurg 1992;121: 627–30.

[44] Kure K, Park YD, Kim TS, et al. Immunohistochemical localization of an HIV epitope in cerebral aneurysmal arteriopathy in pediatric acquired immune deficiency syndrome (AIDS). Pediatr Pathol 1989;9:655–67.

[45] Philippet P, Blanche S, Sebas G, et al. Stroke and cerebral infarcts in children infected with human immunodeficiency virus. Arch Pediatr Adolesc Med 1994;148:965–70.

[46] Sedat J, Alvarez H, Rodesch G, et al. Multifocal cervical fusiform aneurysms in children with immune deficiencies: report of four cases. Interventional Neuroradiology 1999;5:151–6.

[47] Dubrovsky T, Curless R, Scott G, et al. Cerebral aneurysmal arteriopathy in childhood AIDS. Neurology 1998;51:560–5.

[48] Shah SS, Zimmerman RA, Rorke LB, et al. Cerebrovascular complications of HIV in children. AJNR Am J Neuroradiol 1996;17:1913–7.

[49] Park YD, Belman AL, Kim TS. Stroke in pediatric acquired immunodeficiency syndrome. Ann Neurol 1990;28:303–11.

[50] Leroy D, Dompmartin A, Houtteville JP, et al. Aneurysm associated with chronic mucocutaneous candidiasis during long-term therapy with ketoconazole. Dermatologica 1989;178: 43–6.

[51] Groubi M, Dalal I, Nisbet-Brown E, et al. Cerebral vasculitis associated with chronic mucocutaneous candidiasis. J Pediatr 1998;133:571–4.

[52] Campos C, Churojana A, Rodesch G, et al. Multiple intracranial arterial aneurysms: a congenital metameric disease? Interventional Neuroradiology 1998;4:293–9.

[53] Waga S, Tochio H. Intracranial aneurysm associated with moyamoya disease in childhood. Surg Neurol 1985;23:237–43.

[54] Vles JS, Hendriks J, Lodder J, et al. Multiple vertebro-basilar infractions from fibromuscular dysplasia related dissecting aneurysm of the vertebral artery in a child. Neuropediatrics 1990;21: 104–25.

[55] Massimi L, Moret J, Tamburrini G, et al. Dissecting giant vertebro-basilar aneurysms. Childs Nerv Syst 2003;19:204–10.

[56] Ohkuma H, Suzuki S, Shimamura N, et al. Dissecting aneurysms of the middle cerebral artery:

neuroradiological and clinical features. Neuroradiology 2003;45:143–8.

[57] Ohkuma H, Suzuki S, Ogane K. Study group of the association of cerebrovascular disease in Tohoku, Japan 2002: dissecting aneurysms of intracranial carotid circulation. Stroke 33:941–947

[58] Tanabe M, Inoue Y, Hori T. Spontaneous thrombosis of an aneurysm of the middle cerebral artery with subarachnoid hemorrhage in a 6-year-old child. Neurol Res 1991;13:202–4.

[59] Krings T, Piske RL, Lausjaunias PL. Intracranial arterial aneurysm vasculopathies: targeting the outer vessel wall. Neuroradiology 2005;47:931–7.

[60] Lazinski D, Willinsky R, terBrugge KG, et al. Dissecting aneurysms of the posterior cerebral artery: angioarchitecture and a review of the literature. Neuroradiology 2000;42:128–33.

[61] Weil SM, Olivi A, Greiner AL, et al. Multiple intracranial aneurysms in identical twins. Acta Neurochir (Wien) 1988;95:121–5.

[62] Kuchelmeister K, Schulz R, Bergmann M, et al. A probably familial saccular aneurysm of the anterior communicating artery in a neonate. Childs Nerv Syst 1993;9:302–6.

[63] Ronkainen A, Hernesniemi J, Ryynanen M. Familial subarachnoid hemorrhage in east Finland. 1977–1990. Neurosurgery 1993;33:787–97.

[64] De Blasi R, Lasjaunias P, Rodesch G, et al. Endovascular treatment of a ruptured intracranial arterial aneurysm in a 12-year-old child with recessive polycystic kidney disease. Interventional Neuroradiology 1997;3:333–6.

[65] Lapresle J, Lasjaunias P, Verret JM, et al. Anévrysme géant de la carotide intracaverneuse compliqué d'hémorrhagie méningée [Giant aneurysm of the intracavernous carotid, complicated by subarachnoid haemorhage. Emergency treatment by occlusive balloon and thrombosis in situ]. Nouv Presse Med 1979;8:3037–40 [in French].

[66] Higashida RT, Halbach VV, Dowd C, et al. Intracranial aneurysms: interventional neurovascular treatment with detachable balloons. Results in 215 cases. Radiology 1991;178:663–70.

[67] Banna M, Terbrugge K, Lasjaunias P, et al. Embolization of dissecting aneurysms of the petrocavernous segment of the carotid artery. Can Assoc Radiol J 1991;42:265–9.

[68] Numaguchi Y, Peusner P, Rigamonti D, et al. Platinum coil treatment of complex aneurysms of the vertebrobasilar circulation. Neuroradiology 1992;34:252–5.

[69] Al-Qahtani S, Tampieri D, Brassard R, et al. Coil embolization of an aneurysm associated with an infraoptic anterior cerebral artery in a child. AJNR Am J Neuroradiol 2003;24:990–1.

[70] Grosso S, Mostardini R, Venturi C, et al. Recurrent torticollis caused by dissecting vertebral artery aneurysm in a pediatric patient: results of endovascular treatment by use of coil embolization. Case report. Neurosurgery 2002;50:204–7 [discussion: 207–8].

[71] Dorfler A, Wanke I, Wiedemayer H, et al. Endovascular treatment of a giant aneurysm of the internal carotid artery in a child with visual loss: case report. Neuropediatrics 2000;31:151–4.

[72] Sanai N, Quinones-Hinojosa A, Gupta NM, et al. Pediatric intracranial aneurysms: durability of treatment following microsurgical and endovascular management. J Neurosurg 2006; 104(2 Suppl):82–9.

[73] Little JR, Larkins MV, Lüders H, et al. Fusiform basilar artery aneurysm in a 33-month-old child. Neurosurgery 1986;19:631–4.

ELSEVIER
SAUNDERS

NEUROIMAGING
CLINICS
OF NORTH AMERICA

Neuroimag Clin N Am 17 (2007) 165–173

Endovascular Treatment of Hemangiomas

Joon K. Song, MD[a,*], Yasunari Niimi, MD[a,b],
Alejandro Berenstein, MD[a,b]

Hemangiomas are vascular tumors that enlarge through proliferation of endothelial cells. They are the most common tumors of infancy, appearing in as many as 10% to 12% of children under 1 year of age, with double this incidence in preterm infants weighing less than 1000 g [1]. In the children of mothers who have undergone chorionic-villus sampling, the incidence of hemangiomas has been reported to be 10 times higher [2]. Female-to-male predominance is about 4:1.

Most hemangiomas appear in the first 6 weeks of life. Hemangiomas can be seen in the skin in 4% to 10% of Caucasian newborns, and less frequently in non-Caucasians [3,4]. The head and neck regions are involved most frequently (60% of cases), followed by the trunk (25% of cases) and the extremities (15% of cases). Hemangiomas occur as an isolated lesion in 80% of cases, whereas they are multifocal in 20%. Involvement of the liver, gastrointestinal tract, or lungs is common in patients who have multiple cutaneous lesions. Central nervous system involvement is rare, usually associated with the disseminated form, and often lethal.

Despite their benign nature, hemangiomas can cause significant morbidity if not recognized and treated properly. The management of hemangiomas has emerged as interdisciplinary, with endovascular treatment an important component.

Clinical presentation and natural history

At birth, hemangiomas appear as small, pale, or erythematous macules, red spots, ecchymotic-like patches, or telangiectasias. After birth, the lesion is noted to grow and, if superficial, appears more as a bright red, slightly raised, noncompressible plaque lesion (Fig. 1). Less superficial lesions involving the deep dermis or subcutaneous tissue may have minimal, blush-like discoloration, or no skin involvement at all (Fig. 2). Deeper hemangiomas present several months later and are noted only when they produce contour asymmetry. Hemangiomas are characterized by a rapid growth, or proliferative, phase, which may last up to 18 months, at which point growth reaches a plateau. Nearly all

[a] Hyman-Newman Institute for Neurology and Neurosurgery and the Center for Endovascular Surgery, Roosevelt Hospital, 1000 Tenth Avenue, 10th Floor, New York, NY 10019, USA
[b] The Albert Einstein College of Medicine
* Corresponding author. Hyman-Newman Institute for Neurology and Neurosurgery and the Center for Endovascular Surgery, Roosevelt Hospital, 1000 Tenth Avenue, 10th Floor, New York, NY 10019.
E-mail address: jsong@chpnet.org (J.K. Song).

doi:10.1016/j.nic.2007.02.003

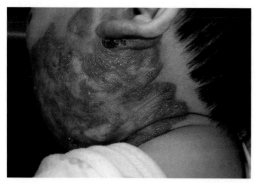

Fig. 1. Superficial facial hemangioma. This 16-month-old female patient has an extensive hemangioma involving the left parotid, cheek, neck, and upper chest.

hemangiomas go through a spontaneous involuting phase. Areas of ulceration or necrosis, with patchy healing, are not infrequent. By 5 years of age, 50% of hemangiomas will have achieved complete involution, and 70% by 7 years of age, with the remaining children showing continued improvement until ages 10 to 12 (Fig. 3) [5]. In approximately one half of children, the skin at that time will appear normal.

Diagnosis

Superficial hemangiomas are easy to diagnose on physical examination because of their characteristic red, raised, strawberry-like appearance. The lesions are soft on palpation and warm to touch, and may be pulsatile, with an audible bruit during the proliferative phase. Deeper lesions with intact overlying skin may be more difficult to diagnose. The

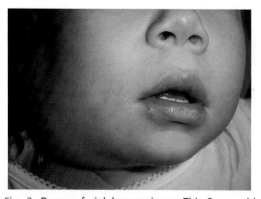

Fig. 2. Deeper facial hemangioma. This 2-year-old female patient has a right parotid hemangioma similar, but smaller, than that in Fig. 1, with no evidence of involution. MR imaging demonstrated this to be a hypervascular lesion with prominent flow voids.

skin color may appear blue because of the presence of dilated draining veins beneath the skin. Other characteristic physical features include a pale halo around the lesion, and superficial telangiectasias. The history of rapid postnatal growth followed by stabilization and involution is helpful in making the diagnosis. Usually, the first sign of the involuting phase is marked by a change from the bright reddish, purplish, or crimson color of the cutaneous component to a grayish, patchy, less intense vascular soft tissue, with decreased or absent pulsations. Involuting lesions have a soft, fatty consistency.

Hemangiomas without skin involvement can be differentiated clinically from malformations because of their rapid proliferation, which is faster than the normal growth of the patient. In infants with large lesions, swelling can be seen, particularly if the hemangioma has large draining veins. An increase in size during crying episodes is more characteristic of a venous malformation. However, in some scalp locations associated with a bone defect or located over a bony suture, pulsatility and a transient increase in size during crying episodes may be noted as well [6].

Although most hemangiomas can be diagnosed clinically, deep lesions require imaging to rule out soft-tissue malignancies and vascular malformations. The hallmark of hemangiomas on imaging is the combination of a homogeneous, solid, parenchymal mass with evidence of increased vascularity, and less frequent high-flow vascular supply and drainage. Ultrasound scanning with Doppler imaging demonstrates the solid parenchymal component with dilated vessels inside and around the lesion. Doppler assessment of the vessels indicates high flow with decreased arterial resistance and increased venous velocity, consistent with microshunting. With involution, the vessels become smaller, and the Doppler flow more normal. CT shows hemangiomas to be similar, or lower in density than surrounding muscle, with uniformly dense contrast enhancement and demonstration of feeding and draining vessels around and below the lesion. During and after involution, subcutaneous lesions appear to have increasing amounts of intralesional fat and smaller vessels, with no associated bone hypertrophy. MR imaging demonstrates a lobulated, parenchymal mass with dilated feeding arteries and draining veins within and around the lesion (Fig. 4). Hemangiomas are iso- or hypointense on T1-weighted sequences, and moderately hyperintense on T2-weighted sequences. They enhance uniformly in the proliferating phase. Gradient sequences confirm the high-flow vessels within and around the solid mass. Analysis of associated deep and intracranial lesions, if suspected,

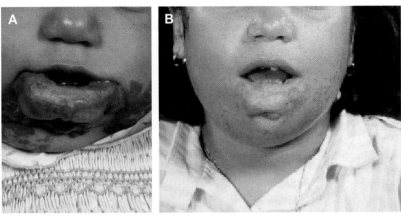

Fig. 3. Sequence of hemangioma involution.

makes MR imaging particularly helpful under these circumstances. MR angiography is of no particular value at present.

Angiography is not needed for diagnosis. When performed at the time of planned endovascular embolization, it demonstrates dilated feeding arteries, organized gland-like arterial angioarchitecture with a dense parenchymal blush, and drainage into dilated adjacent veins (Fig. 5). Venous filling may be very rapid, indicating arteriovenous shunting. It is sometimes difficult to distinguish hemangiomas from hypervascular soft-tissue tumors, which tend to have less well defined margins and irregular vessels, with signs of encasement and neovascularity.

Pathology

Advances in the biological characterization of vascular lesions have increased our understanding of hemangiomas. The work of Mulliken and Glowacki in 1982 [7] provided the basis for these changes. Mulliken and Glowacki, using tissue culture, histochemical, and electron microscopic studies, classified vascular lesions on the basis of endothelial behavior. They divided vascular lesions into two groups: hemangiomas and vascular malformations. Vascular malformations are lesions of defective vessel remodeling without evidence of cellular proliferation, although an active role is played by certain growth factors. Histologic findings in vascular

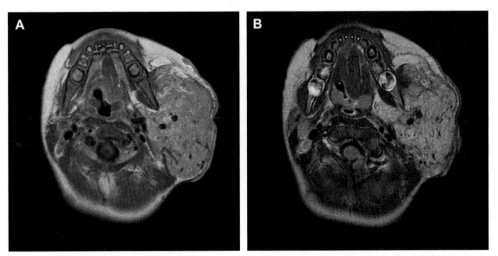

Fig. 4. MR imaging demonstrates a lobulated parenchymal mass with dilated feeding arteries and draining veins both within and around the lesion. Hemangiomas are iso- or hypointense on T1-weighted sequences and enhance densely postcontrast (*A*), and moderately hyperintense on T2-weighted sequences (*B*). Note flow voids from vessels within the lesion.

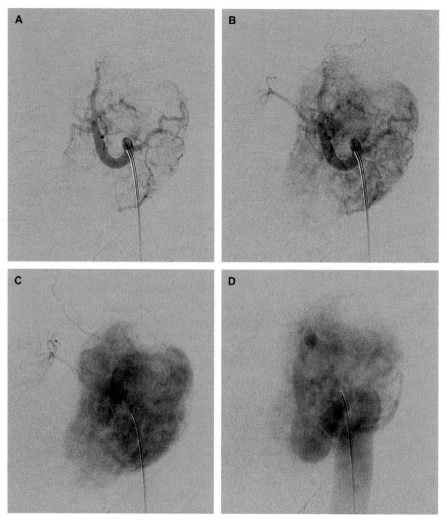

Fig. 5. Angiogram of parotid hemangioma, sequential from early arterial to late venous phase (*A–D*). From internal maxillary artery injection when performed at the time of planned endovascular embolization, it demonstrates dilated feeding arteries, organized gland-like arterial angioarchitecture with a dense parenchymal blush, and drainage into dilated adjacent veins. (Same patient as in Fig. 2.)

malformations relate to the channel abnormalities present, and the endothelium may show qualitative changes without evidence of increased cell turnover. Hemangiomas show endothelial hyperplasia and turnover, with an elevated mast cell population in the basement membrane leading to a rapid proliferative phase, then to a stable plateau phase, followed by an involution phase. Histologic findings in hemangiomas include plump, rapidly dividing endothelial cells with lumina of various sizes, pericytes, and multilaminated basement membranes. During involution, mitotic activity decreases, mast cells appear and subsequently disappear, and endothelial cells drop out (apoptosis) and are replaced progressively by deposits of perivascular and intralobular fibrous and adipose tissue. Nothing in the vessels or stroma has been found that would predict

involution. Possible mechanisms of involution include occlusion of the vascular bed by endothelial cellular proliferation or induced by humoral factors. Histologically, during involution, there is a lack of thrombosis or infarction.

An important addition to our understanding is the recent identification of various cellular markers in proliferating hemangiomas, including proliferating cell nuclear antigen, type IV collagenase, vascular endothelial growth factor, basic fibroblast growth factor (bFGF), E-selectin, and urokinase [8]. These markers are absent in vascular malformations. Hemangiomas overexpress the angiogenic proteins bFGF and vascular endothelial growth factor during the proliferating phase, and preliminary data indicate that the diagnosis of hemangioma can be supported, and the results of therapy monitored, by measuring bFGF levels in the urine [8]. Cellular proliferation in hemangiomas is inhibited by interferon-a. In 2000, North and colleagues [9] made the observation that hemangiomas are always positive for a specific immunohistochemical marker, not linked to mitotic activity, which reliably distinguishes endothelial cells of juvenile hemangiomas at all stages of their evolution, in both proliferative and involutive phases. Infantile hemangiomas display positive immunoreactivity for glucose transporter GLUT1, Lewis Y (LeY) antigen, and Fc gamma receptor II (FcγRII), all placenta-associated antigens found in the endothelium only at sites of blood tissue barriers, such as neural tissue and placenta, but not seen in any other vascular tissue from tumors, malformations, or granulations [10,11].

Although not proven, given this immunophenotypic pattern and the presence of hemangiomas in the perinatal period, it has been postulated that hemangiomas may represent systemic metastasis from placental cells, or from angioblasts aberrantly switched toward the placental endothelium phenotype, either by somatic mutation or abnormal local inductive influences [9,10]. Another theory suggests that the apparent random distribution of hemangiomas is not random, that the more frequent distribution in the head, neck, back of the torso, and other locations seems to correlate with early cells of common origin, such as neural crest or dorsal mesoderm cells, and, therefore, with potentially similar vulnerability. During the perinatal period, the placenta releases regulators of angiogenesis. One such factor is Flt-1 (sFlt-1), a potent inhibitor of angiogenesis present in the placenta and amniotic fluid that helps regulate angiogenesis and is found in a high concentration toward the end of gestation [12]. One may postulate that if no longer under the regulation of such angiogenesis inhibitors, a single "target" (single hemangiomas) or multiple "targets" (multiple hemangiomas) in the immediate perinatal period may result in unrepressed proliferation, or hemangiogenesis. Recently, based on X-chromosome inactivation studies, Boye and colleagues [13] reported that endothelial cells of hemangiomas are clonal. Blei and colleagues [14] and Walter and colleagues [15] reported the rare association of familial occurrences.

The distribution of head and neck hemangiomas does not appear to be random [16]. Head and neck hemangiomas have two patterns of growth: a more prevalent focal mass (three times more common) and a diffuse, plaque-like lesion. They occur near lines of mesenchymal or mesenchymal-ectodermal embryonic fusion [16]. The most frequent location for focal hemangiomas is the midcheek, followed by the lateral upper lip and then the upper eyelid.

Diffuse hemangiomas show a more segmental distribution, such as frontonasal, maxillary, and mandibular, in relatively equal proportions.

Complications

Approximately 20% of hemangiomas are associated with symptoms that may require treatment [17]. It has been estimated that 1% of hemangiomas are life threatening. Dermatologic complications, manifesting as hypertrophy of the epidermis and subcutaneous tissues, can result in ulceration and are seen in up to 5% of hemangiomas [18]. Secondary infection and bleeding may result, before or during the period of ulceration. These complications are also known to de-accelerate the regression of the proliferative phenomenon. The cutaneous extension of superficial capillary hemangiomas can leave visible skin scars, even after complete regression. Ulcerations may be destructive, and may result in destruction of facial features, particularly in the lip and the tip of the nose (Cyrano nose hemangioma).

Additional complications can occur including congestive heart failure, seen primarily in hepatic or pelvic lesions [6,19], and hemorrhage. Congestive heart failure is seldom seen in head and neck hemangiomas. Usually, hemorrhage is limited, unless associated with a hemangioendothelioma with a consumption coagulopathy, as seen in Kasabach-Merritt syndrome. In rare cases, significant bleeding can occur without a coagulopathy, which is mechanical in nature, such as in the folds of a rapidly proliferating lesion.

Focal mass effect may be important in periorbital, nose, mouth, and airway locations. It may have immediate consequences, such as compromise to vital functions, or delayed consequences, which may result in either functional symptoms (blindness or various optical abnormalities) or dysmorphic symptoms (induced mandibular growth alteration in the nose, lip, or earlobe). The psychologic impact of cosmetic impairment in infants and children with hemangiomas, particularly in the head and neck, is important to consider.

Indications

A few management principles have emerged with the better understanding of hemangiomas and the emergence of multidisciplinary teams that specialize in maxillo-facial treatment in the pediatric population. Knowledge of the natural history of hemangiomas is imperative in determining the proper course of treatment. If a good early surgical excision is not possible, observation is recommended because most hemangiomas in the head and neck invariably involute. It appears that in most cases, a surgical excision is possible [20] that will permit the child to reach a normal appearance during the critical formative years. Early intervention, pioneered by Waner and Suen [20], is gaining wider acceptance.

Treatment

Medical

Corticosteroids

Zarem and Edgerton's [21] discovery of the effect of oral corticosteroid on hemangiomas in 1967 was fortuitous. These researchers observed the resolution of a facial hemangioma after administering systemic corticosteroid for the treatment of hemangioma-associated thrombocytopenia. Steroids are effective mainly in the early, active, proliferating phase, which occurs in the first 6 to 8 months. All routes of administration have been implemented. The definitive mechanism of action is not clear, but proposed explanations include sensitization of the hemangiomatous vasculature to circulating endogenous vasoconstrictors [22]. Sasaki and colleagues [23] described the influence of corticosteroids on hormone receptors in hemangiomas. Folkman and coworkers [24] reported that cortisone inhibited angiogenesis in the presence of heparin. Reports of successful response to systemic corticosteroids treatment vary from 30% [25,26] to 93% [20].

Potential known complications of corticosteroid therapy include immunosuppression, with increased frequency of childhood infections [27]. Cushingoid changes, failure to thrive, increased appetite, and irritability are reversible [28]. In an effort to overcome the systemic side effects or the risk of intralesional injections, clobetasol cream, a potent topical steroid, has been used, as in the treatment of periorbital hemangiomas. Systemic or local steroid treatment is not always effective in capillary hemangiomas [26], with the exception of Kasabach Merritt syndrome, and some rebound growth may be observed after discontinuation. However, it may take 1 or 2 weeks to observe a response, occasionally a too-rapid involution with necrosis and ulceration can occur, leading to considerable problems of reconstruction. Rebound and intolerance should prompt a change in treatment.

Interferon-alpha 2a, vincristine, and others

Interferon alpha 2a, originally developed as an antiviral agent, was noted to have an unexpected effect on Kaposi's sarcoma (a vascular tumor) during treatment trials in patients who had AIDS, which led to the discovery that this agent also acted as an antiangiogenic drug. Further studies revealed that interferon inhibits the advancement of capillary endothelium in vitro and angiogenesis in mice. Subsequent to these discoveries, the role of interferon in treating life-threatening hemangiomas has been controversial, with limited acceptability.

Important side effects of interferon therapy include elevation of liver enzymes and irreversible neurotoxicity [29], including an unacceptably high incidence (approximately 20%–25%) of severe spastic diplegia, presenting sometimes months after treatment with interferon, and usually irreversible. Therefore, with the exception of severe, bilateral, vision-threatening orbital hemangiomas, or those with intracranial extension, or life-threatening lesions that fail to respond to steroid treatment without a good surgical or endovascular option, the current recommendation appears to be to avoid interferon.

Vincristine has been shown to be effective for some refractory cases of hemangioma. However, because of serious and sometimes delayed neurologic complications, this therapy is no longer recommended for hemangiomas.

Aminocaproic acid has been used in some patients, but it is also not an innocuous drug, and is reserved for cases with consumption coagulopathy. Streptokinase, heparin, and aspirin have been used with mixed results.

Radiation

Hemangiomas are responsive to radiation therapy, but this modality currently is not favored because of its long-term side effects (malignancy, regional growth impairment, and scarring).

Surgery, Laser, and Embolization

Waner and Suen [20] have advocated early intervention with surgery, laser, intralesional laser, and embolization in selected cases, even in the proliferative stage, to prevent disfiguration or subsequent mutilating interventions. In lesions that are hypervascular and do not flatten or disappear after embolization, surgery may achieve excellent results.

Almost all forms of medical laser have been used to treat hemangiomas. In superficial telangiectasias associated with a regressing hemangioma, pulse-dye photocoagulation should be used with caution to avoid cutaneous scarring [30]. Nd:YAG laser results have been more dramatic, but are associated with a much higher rate of complication, including delayed healing and permanent scarring. Carbon dioxide laser is more efficacious as an incisional and coagulating tool, as opposed to an ablative instrument. Waner and Suen [20] reported promising results using a carbon dioxide laser for resurfacing atrophic changes of involutional hemangiomas.

The flashlamp–pumped dye laser (also called pulsed-dye laser and tunable-dye laser) [20,31] is regarded now as the laser of choice for hemangiomas because its wavelength can be modified. For hemangiomas, the wavelength is set between 585 and 600 nm (yellow light). A longer wavelength results in deeper penetration, but carries with it an increased risk of hypopigmentation. Pulse duration is another critical factor in the use of this type of laser. Longer exposure time addresses larger vessels, but, at the same time, increases thermal damage to surrounding tissue.

Arterial embolization employing microparticles or liquid embolic agents such as N-butyl cyanoacrylate (NBCA) can produce significant ischemia and necrosis within the tumor, which can expedite involution. At present, the authors use embolization preoperatively in hypervascular lesions (parotid or "beard" distribution lesions), mostly in young children where blood volume is limited (see Fig. 5). They have observed accelerated involution that is shifting their therapeutic strategy to liquid (NBCA) embolization followed by surgical excision (Fig. 6). This method is also indicated in the treatment of life-threatening hemangiomas, where drug treatment has failed, or where mass reduction is required rapidly, before the anticipated response to medical therapy, and in cardiac failure. Embolization of at least 70% of the arterial supply is necessary to produce a significant clinical response [32]. The mass will decrease rapidly in size (in 2–4 days), and then stabilize and likely follow a spontaneous favorable regression course.

Several side effects of embolization are noted. Pain is usually absent, but it may be noted if normal tissues has been embolized together with the hemangioma.

Arterial-arterial anastomoses with the intracranial circulation are open in babies and children. The hypervascularity of hemangiomas produces a "sump" effect toward the hemangioma, maintaining a craniofugal flow toward the lesion, which makes the anastomoses invisible during the pre-embolization work-up in the external carotid branches. As the embolization progresses and the flow in the lesion diminishes, a reversal of flow through anastomoses can occur; therefore, continuous fluoroscopic monitoring and control angiography are necessary.

Volume overload in children with large hemangiomas represents a technical challenge because it requires multiple arterial feeder embolizations and many particle injections with contrast material. Even in dealing with infants who weigh more than 5 kg, it is necessary to be careful with the number of injections during embolization to avoid the use of large amounts of contrast material. The authors, therefore, prefer liquid embolic agents, because they require significantly less contrast and radiation. If an important anastomosis is seen or suspected, this territory can be protected safely with an endovascular liquid coil.

Separate supply from multiple sources constitutes a frequent challenge because numerous selective catheterizations of various branches will be necessary, each of them contributing only a small amount to the overall supply. Multiple sessions may be necessary in such circumstances, and staging the procedure will permit a larger contrast material load.

Direct percutaneous puncture intralesional embolization under fluoroscopic monitoring can be performed with ethanol (Fig. 7) or glue, alone or in combination with transarterial embolization. Although better penetration usually can be achieved by direct percutaneous puncture, caution is important, mostly when using cytotoxic liquids such as alcohol, as one must ensure intravascular position

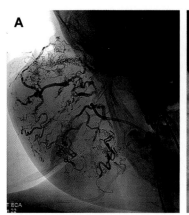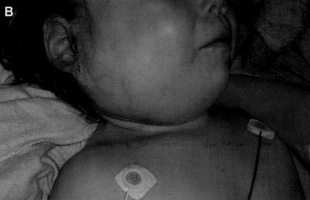

Fig. 6. Glue casts (*A*) are shown for same patient as in Fig. 2. Following surgical excision, results are excellent (*B*).

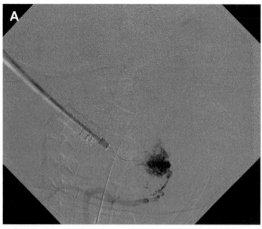
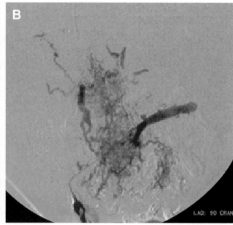

Fig. 7. Direct percutaneous puncture intralesional embolization under fluoroscopic monitoring can be done with ethanol (*A*) or glue (*B*), alone or in combination with transarterial embolization. Intravascular position is paramount for direct percutaneous puncture intralesional embolization.

into the minute channels representing the vascular bed of these proliferative lesions. In most instances, injections involve the interstitial space instead of the vascular bed. Such an approach should be reserved for urgent cases in which patients fail to respond to medical therapy, or when surgery is not considered to be an effective option and arterial embolization treatment is unsuccessful.

More recently, the use of direct puncture using bleomycin appears encouraging, but the authors do not have experience with this agent [33].

References

[1] Amir J, Metzker A, Krikler R, et al. Strawberry hemangioma in preterm infants. Pediatr Dermatol 1986;3:331–2.

[2] Burton BKl. An increased incidence of hemangiomas in infants born following chorionic sampling. Prenat Diagn 1995;15:209–14.

[3] Jacobs AH, Walton RG. The incidence of birthmarks in the neonate. Pediatrics 1976;58:218–22.

[4] Hidano A, Nakajima S. Earliest features of the strawberry mark in the newborn. Br J Dermatol 1972;87:138–44.

[5] Bingham HG. Predicting the course of a congenital hemangioma. Plast Reconstr Surg 1979;63:161–6.

[6] Martinez-Perez D, Fein NA, Boon LM, et al. Not all hemangiomas look like strawberries: uncommon presentation of the most common tumor of infancy. Pediatr Dermatol 1995;12:1–6.

[7] Mulliken JB, Glowacki J. Hemangiomas and vascular malformation in children: a classification based on endothelial characteristics. Plast Reconstr Surg 1982;69:412–22.

[8] Takahashi K, Mulliken JB, Kozakewich HP, et al. Cellular markers that distinguish the phases of hemangioma during infancy and childhood. J Clin Invest 1994;93(6):2357–64.

[9] North PE, Waner M, Mizeracki A, et al. GLUT1: a newly discovered immunochemical marker for juvenile hemangiomas. Hum Pathol 2000; 31:11–22.

[10] North PE, Waner M, Mizeracki A, et al. A unique microvascular phenotype shared by juvenile hemangiomas and human placenta. Arch Dermatol 2001;137:559–70.

[11] North P, Waner M, Brodsky M. Guest editorial. Are infantile hemangiomas of placental origin? Ophthalmology 2002;109(4):633–4.

[12] Clark DE, Smith SK, He Y, et al. A vascular growth is produced by the human placenta and released into the maternal circulation. Biol Reprod 1998;59:1540–8.

[13] Boye E, Yu Y, Paranya G, et al. Clonality and altered behavior of endothelial cells from hemangiomas. J Clin Invest 2001;107:745–52.

[14] Blei F, Walter J, Orlow SJ, et al. Familial segregation of hemangiomas and vascular malformations as an autosomal dominant trait. Arch Dermatol 1998;134:718–22.

[15] Walter JW, Blei F, Anderson JL, et al. Genetic mapping of a novel familial form of infantile hemangioma. Am J Med Genet 1999;82: 77–83.

[16] Waner M, North PE, Scherer KA, et al. The nonrandom distribution of facial hemangiomas. Arch Dermatol 2003;139:869–75.

[17] Enjolras O, Riche MC, Merland JJ, et al. Management of alarming hemangiomas in infancy: a review of 25 cases. Pediatrics 1990;85(4):491–8.

[18] Margileth AM, Museles M. Cutaneous hemangiomas in children: diagnosis and conservative management. JAMA 1965;194:523.

[19] Boon LM, Enjolras O, Mulliken JB. Congenital hemangiomas: evidence of accelerated involution. J Pediatr 1996;128:329–35.

[20] Waner M, Suen JY. Treatment options for the management of hemangiomas. In: Waner M, Suen JY, editors. Hemangiomas and vascular

malformations of the head and neck. New York: Wiley-Liss; 1999. p. 233–61.

[21] Zarem HA, Edgerton MT. Induced resolution of cavernous hemangiomas following prednisone therapy. Plast Reconstr Surg 1967;39:76–83.

[22] Edgerton MT. The treatment of hemangiomas: with special reference to the role of steroid therapy. Ann Surg 1976;183:517–32.

[23] Sasaki GH, Pang CY, Wittliff JL. Pathogenesis and treatment of infant strawberry hemangiomas: clinical and in-vitro studies of hormonal effects. Plast Reconstr Surg 1984;73:359–70.

[24] Folkman J, Langer R, Linhart RJ, et al. Angiogenesis inhibition and tumor regression caused by heparin and heparin fragments in the presence of cortisone. Science 1983;221:719–25.

[25] Bartoshesky L, Bull M, Feingold M. Corticosteroid treatment of cutaneous hemangiomas: how effective? Clin Pediatr 1978;17:625–38.

[26] Haik BG, Jakobiec FA, Jones IS. Capillary hemangioma of the lids and orbit: an analysis of the clinical features and therapeutic result in 101 cases. Ophthalmology 1979;86:762–92.

[27] Gunn T, Reece E, Metrakos K, et al. Depressed T Cell following neonatal steroid treatment. Pediatrics 1981;6:61–7.

[28] Sadan N, Wolach B. Treatment of hemangiomas of infants with high doses of prednisone. J Pediatr 1996;128(1):141–6.

[29] Egbert JE, Nelson SC. Neurologic toxicity associated with alfa-interferon treatment of capillary hemangiomas. J AAPOS 1997;1(4):190.

[30] Mulliken JB. A plea for a biological approach to hemangiomas of infancy [editorial]. Arch Dermatol 1991;127:243–4.

[31] Geronemus RG, Ashinoff R. Capillary hemangiomas and treatment with the flash lamp–pumped dye Laser. Arch Dermatol 1991;127:202–5.

[32] Lasjuanias P, ter Brugge KG, Berenstein A. Surgical neuroangiography, vol. 3, clinical and interventional aspects in children. 2nd edition. Berlin Heidelberg: Springer-Verlag; 2006.

[33] Pienaar C, Graham R, Geldenhuys S, et al. Related articles, Intralesional bleomycin for the treatment of hemangiomas. Plast Reconstr Surg 2006;117(1):221–6.

NEUROIMAGING
CLINICS
OF NORTH AMERICA

Neuroimag Clin N Am 17 (2007) 175–187

Arterial Ischemic Stroke in Children

Tali Jonas Kimchi, MD[a,b,*], Ronit Agid, MD[b],
Seon-Kyu Lee, MD, PhD[b], Karel G. Ter Brugge, MD[b]

Stroke in children is relatively rare. Isolated cases of stroke in the pediatric population were documented in the eighteenth and nineteenth century, but no significant epidemiologic data became available until the late 1970s [1]. Most reports in the past focused on the underlying pathologies that can occur in children presenting with a stroke, and few dealt with the outcome of stroke in the various age groups and how treatment might affect them. In fact, the treatment of stroke in children has mainly been geared toward management of the underlying causes.

Advances in the clinical recognition and radiographic diagnosis of ischemic stroke have increased the frequency of the diagnosis in infants and children and have raised the need for immediate therapy including reperfusion therapy and brain protection. Few reports have dealt with the active treatment of acute stroke in children. No randomized control trials have been done other than studies in children with sickle cell disease and adults,

which are not directly applicable to the general pediatric population with a stroke. The lack of published clinical trials and of experience in treating a large number of cases has resulted in a significant challenge for clinicians.

A vast amount of data has recently become available through basic research and neuroimaging techniques shedding new light on the chain of events that occur in ischemic stroke in animal models and in the adult population. Whether this new information can also be applied to the pediatric population remains to be seen, but it is likely that the active management of children with acute ischemic stroke in the near future will include brain protection, brain reperfusion, and prevention measures.

Epidemiology

Vascular occlusive disease is increasingly seen in infants and children. Two population-based studies in the United States have indicated that the

[a] Division of Neuroradiology, Department of Medical Imaging, Sheba Medical Center, Ramat-Gan, Israel
[b] Division of Neuroradiology, Toronto Western Hospital, Department of Medical Imaging, University Health Network (UHN), University of Toronto, Toronto, Ontario, Canada
* Corresponding author. Division of Neuroradiology, Department of Medical Imaging, Sheba Medical Center, Ramat-Gan, Israel.
E-mail address: tali.jonaskimchi@gmail.com (T.J. Kimchi).

1052-5149/07/$ – see front matter © 2007 Elsevier Inc. All rights reserved.   doi:10.1016/j.nic.2007.02.007
neuroimaging.theclinics.com

incidence rate of ischemic and hemorrhagic stroke is 2.52 cases per 100,000 population per year [1] and the rate of ischemic stroke 1.2 cases per 100,000 population per year [2]. The incidence varies in children with different ethnic backgrounds. Based on prospectively collected data from 1985 to 1993 in France, the incidence of ischemic stroke was 8 cases per 100,000 population and the incidence of hemorrhagic stroke 5 cases per 100,000 population [3]. These data were for children less than 16 years of age. Sixty-one percent of the cases were ischemic strokes and 39% were hemorrhagic. In the Canadian Pediatric Ischemic Stroke Registry, 820 children were identified with ischemic stroke aged from birth to 18 years, yielding an incidence of 3.3 cases per 100,000 children per year. Arterial ischemic stroke (AIS) constituted 80% of the cases [4]. A study performed in the North American population based on telephone consultation service showed that 64% of cases were ischemic stroke and 36% sinovenous thrombosis. That study also demonstrated a mean age of 6.2 years. The most affected age group comprised persons from birth to 3 years of age, and neonates comprised 16% of patients. The rate of male gender was 54% [5].

Clinical presentation

The clinical presentation of ischemic stroke in the pediatric population is age related. Neonates with AIS tend to present with convulsions and lethargy. They rarely, if ever, present with an appreciable focal neurologic deficit in the acute phase. The neurologic deficit slowly becomes apparent over the next few months to year (Fig. 1) [6]. Delayed presentation of a neurologic deficit such as decreased hand use occurred in 18 of 22 patients with presumed pre- or perinatal AIS. All of these patients were considered neurologically normal until at least 2 months of age. All 22 patients had some weakness on longer follow-up, and 12 developed permanent signs of speech, cognitive, or behavioral deficits. Five had persistent seizures [7]. The late symptoms can cause delayed diagnosis in this age group.

Infants tend to present with pathologically early hand preference as a sign of previous stroke. The actual time of onset of the stroke often cannot be determined [8]. In fact, the evolution is often similar to that in patients whose strokes are identified during the perinatal period. Sometimes, older infants and toddlers present with abrupt onset of hemiparesis, facial droop, or difficulty in moving one of the extremities [4]. The clinical presentation not infrequently consists of fever, convulsion, and coma.

Presentation of stroke in later childhood is typically an acute neurologic deficit, usually hemiparesis (Fig. 2). Subtle signs such as speech or visual disturbances, headache, or sensory deficits can also be part of the presentation. Seizures can accompany the stroke in 50% of cases [4]. In a study recently published in Turkey, 79 patients presented with a stroke. Fifty-seven had acute ischemic stroke; the mean age of that group was 29.6 months. Thirty-nine of the patients presented with hemiparesis. Eleven patients had seizures, and five had altered mental status [9].

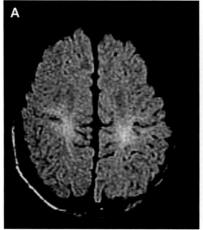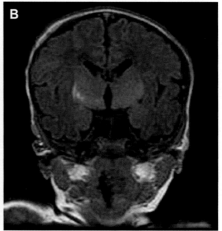

Fig. 1. Four-week-old neonate with progressive neurologic deficits. MR imaging demonstrates the typical findings of hypoxic-ischemic perinatal encephalopathy. (*A*) Diffusion-weighted image shows the typical peri-rolandic ischemic changes as hyperintense signal. (*B*) Coronal T1-weighted image demonstrates hyperintense signal in the basal ganglia.

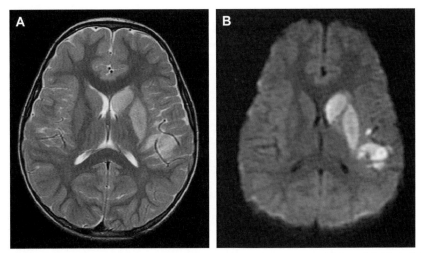

Fig. 2. MR imaging 1 day after onset of right-sided weakness in a 3-year-old boy. (*A*) T2-weighted image. (*B*) Diffusion-weighted image demonstrates subcortical and basal-ganglia infarcts. (*From* Berenstein A, Lasjaunias PL, TerBrugge KG, editors. Surgical neuro-angiography, vol. 3. Berlin, Heidelberg, New York: Springer-Verlag; 2006; with permission.)

Etiology

The causes of ischemic stroke in children are varied and differ significantly from the underlying causes in adults. In the majority of children (80%), a specific etiologic cause for the stroke can be found. In pediatric AIS, arteriopathies, cardiac disease, and prothrombotic disorders are the most commonly recognized risk factors (Fig. 3).

Different causes will be found according to the geography, including sickle cell disease in North America and infectious causes in India or sub-Saharan countries. Etiologies are sometimes intricate and their mechanisms combined. All children have some sort of infection every 6 months and are exposed daily to more or less benign trauma while playing. Post infectious, post traumatic etiologies are often discussed, such as dissection, concentric proliferation, and emboli. Any combination of these entities can be seen in stroke in children.

The etiologies of AIS in childhood are often multifactorial and different from those in adults, in whom arteriosclerotic disease is the single most common cause. Extensive investigations need to be conducted in children to facilitate understanding the pathogenesis. The following constitute some of the examinations performed to determine the cause of stroke in children:

Blood samples, including a count, serum electrolytes, C-reactive protein or erythrocyte

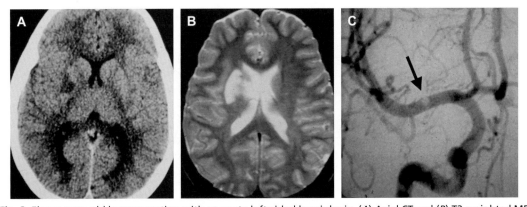

Fig. 3. Eleven-year-old boy presenting with an acute left-sided hemiplegia. (*A*) Axial CT and (*B*) T2-weighted MR image demonstrate a right-sided, basal ganglia infarct. (*C*) Anteroposterior view of a right internal carotid arteriogram shows a filling defect (*arrow*) in the M1 segment of the right middle cerebral artery. This finding is compatible with an embolus of cardiac origin in view of the patient's intermittent cardiac arrhythmia. The embolus is occluding the origin of lateral lenticulo-striate perforators. (*From* Berenstein A, Lasjaunias PL, TerBrugge KG, editors. Surgical neuro-angiography, vol. 3. Berlin, Heidelberg, New York: Springer-Verlag; 2006; with permission.)

sedimentation rate, coagulation times, and fibrinogen titer

Blood samples for measurement of triglycerides and cholesterol, amino acid chromatography, lactates, protein C, protein S, antithrombin III, and antiphospholipid antibodies

Urine samples for amino acid chromatography and organic acid chromatography

Cerebrospinal fluid (CSF) examination for cell count and protein titration, titer of viral antibodies in serum and CSF, or complement and polymerase chain reaction for varicella zoster virus DNA

An echocardiogram, standard electroencephalogram (ECG), prolonged (24-hour) ECG recording, CT, MR imaging, and digital subtraction arteriography

Cardiac disorders

The most common identifiable cause of childhood stroke is congenital heart disease. The most common underlying cardiac conditions are Fallot's tetralogy and transposition of the great vessels. Emboli from the heart or from the periphery through a right-to-left shunt are significant causes of ischemic stroke in the pediatric population (Fig. 4). Thrombi can form on prosthetic cardiac valves and represent another important cause of cerebral emboli. Stroke can also happen at the time of cardiac procedures (catheterization or surgery) [10].

Kaplan and colleagues [11] reported the rate of AIS after cardiac catheterization to be 1.9 cases per 1000 procedures and the rate after surgery 1.0 cases per 1000 procedures.

Genetic diseases involving the cardiovascular system and causing stroke are rare but should be suspected in certain cases [12]. One example is hereditary hemorrhagic telangiectasia (Osler-Weber-Rendu disease), which can be associated with early stroke (neonatal or infant) secondary to a pulmonary arteriovenous fistula [13].

Establishing the etiologic cause of an embolic stroke is not based exclusively on transthoracic cardiac ultrasound. Transesophageal ultrasound can be used in young children to reveal a thrombus or a patent foramen ovale with paradoxical emboli. Because artificially induced dysrhythmia represents a risk factor for embolic stroke, Holter monitoring and other studies are required to rule it out. As a rule, the younger the child, the more likely congenital heart disease will be the cause, in particular before the age of 2 years.

Vasculopathy

Fever or evidence of infection is common in children presenting with cerebral infarction. Bacterial or viral meningitis can be responsible for an infectious type of arteritis resulting in stroke in children [14]. Chicken pox occurred in the 12 months before the onset of symptoms in 31% of children (among 70 children) presenting with AIS who

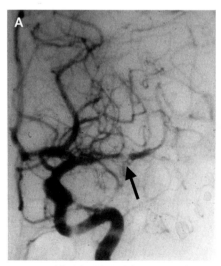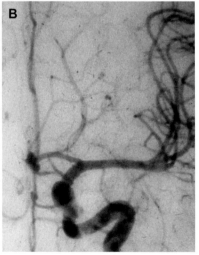

Fig. 4. Fourteen-year-old girl with sudden onset of right hemiplegia and aphasia. The girl has congenital heart disease, cardiac valve protrusion, and arrhythmias. (*A*) Anteroposterior view of left internal carotid angiogram demonstrates a filling defect and near-complete occlusion of the M1 segment of the left middle cerebral artery (*arrow*). (*B*) Angiogram 3 months later demonstrates complete resolution of the finding. (*From* Berenstein A, Lasjaunias PL, TerBrugge KG, editors. Surgical neuro-angiography, vol. 3. Berlin, Heidelberg, New York: Springer-Verlag; 2006; with permission.)

were aged 6 months to 10 years in comparison with 9% of the population [15]. Stroke has been described as a rare complication in children infected with HIV, occurring in about 1% of affected children, although autopsy evidence of infection has been documented in 10% to 30% [16].

Transient cerebral arteriopathy is characterized by a temporary attack on the cerebral arterial wall and accounted for 26% of childhood strokes in Sebire's series [17]. This arteriopathy is presumed to be secondary to an inflammatory process, possibly triggered by an infectious agent such as varicella zoster virus or bacterial agents (Fig. 5) [18,19]. One of the most striking features of this arteriopathy is the transient action of the pathologic process. This transient nature has been demonstrated angiographically by repeated examinations showing, often after initial worsening, regression or stabilization of arterial lesions and clinically by long-term follow-up showing a lack of late recurrence. This acute regressive arteriopathy might represent an important part of ischemic strokes in childhood [17]. The angiographic appearance characterized by focal or segmental stenosis and tail-like occlusions does not suggest an embolic or a thrombotic process but is consistent with abnormalities of the arterial wall (Fig. 6). The pathophysiology of such arterial lesions cannot be established on an angiographic basis. The acute and regressive course is consistent with an acute process such as arteritis, dissection, or vasospasm. The lack of anamnestic events (eg, drug absorption, trauma, or meningeal hemorrhage) and the persistence of arterial lesions make the hypothesis of a vasospasm or dissection unlikely.

Noninfectious vasculitis such as periarteritis nodosa and systemic lupus erythematosus, which are known to be associated with cerebral infarction in adults, rarely cause stroke in children. Isolated angiitis of the central nervous system in children is even more rare, with only 10 cases reported [20]. Takayasu's disease, an arteritis that mainly involves the aorta and its branches, is characterized by hypertension, absent pulses, and vascular bruits. Stroke occurs in 5% to 10% of patients. The disease most commonly affects females between 15 and 20 years of age but has also been reported in infants [21].

Dissection

In Ganesan and colleagues' [22] series investigating risk factors in 212 children with AIS, 185 patients had arterial imaging (87%). A total of 147 patients had vascular abnormalities, including occlusion and narrowing of vessels, dissections, and moyamoya disease. Arterial dissections were demonstrated in 14 cases. Another series reported dissections in 20% of patients with AIS [23].

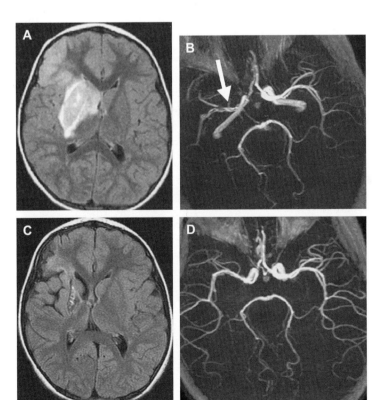

Fig. 5. Seven-year-old girl, 3 months post varicella zoster infection. (A) Flair and (B) MR angiogram images demonstrate an infarct in the basal ganglia on the right with narrowing and irregularity along the right M1 segment (arrow). (C, D) The same MR imaging sequences after 1 year demonstrate normal evolution of the stroke with brain tissue volume loss and resolution of the findings on MR angiography in keeping with transient cerebral angiopathy. (From Berenstein A, Lasjaunias PL, TerBrugge KG, editors. Surgical neuro-angiography, vol. 3. Berlin, Heidelberg, New York: Springer-Verlag; 2006; with permission.)

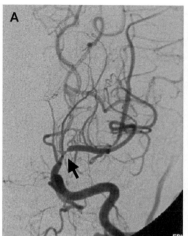
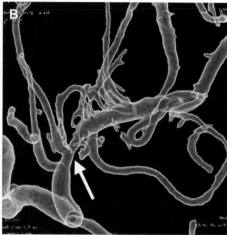

Fig. 6. Five-year-old boy presenting with sudden right-sided hemiplegia following herpes zoster infection. (*A, B*) Cerebral angiogram of the left internal carotid artery in (*A*) anteroposterior view and (*B*) transparent three-dimensional reconstruction in oblique view demonstrate narrowing of the internal carotid artery termination (*arrows*) suggestive of post infectious transient cerebral angiopathy. (*From* Berenstein A, Lasjaunias PL, TerBrugge KG, editors. Surgical neuro-angiography, vol. 3. Berlin, Heidelberg, New York: Springer-Verlag; 2006; with permission.)

Schievink and colleagues [24] described 18 children less than 18 years of age with arterial dissections. Eleven dissections involved the cervical segments, and seven were intracranial. Intracranially, only the anterior circulation was involved. In the neck, the carotid was involved more commonly than the vertebral artery. All of the patients had cerebral or retinal symptoms. In a meta-analysis investigating dissections in the pediatric population, 118 patients were identified. All of the patients had evidence of cerebral ischemia. There was male predominance, and headache was reported in 50% of the cases. Sixty percent of anterior circulation cases were intracranial. It seems that the traumatic dissections are dominantly extracranial and the nontraumatic dissections intracranial. The most common location in the posterior circulation was the vertebral artery at the C1-C2 level (Fig. 7) [25]. In the Canadian pediatric stroke registry, 7.5% of AIS patients had a dissection. Fifty percent had a history of trauma. Clinical features included headache (44%), focal deficits (87.5%), altered consciousness (25%), and seizures (12.5%). Seventy-five percent of the cases had extracranial involvement [26].

Clinical findings in dissection are characterized by a higher mean age, male dominance, and previous head or neck trauma (1–7 days before). The onset of neurologic symptoms may be delayed by hours or days after the injury and may have a sudden onset or a stepwise progression. Horner's syndrome raises the possibility of ipsilateral adventitial carotid artery involvement. Strokes are preceded by headache in most cases. Emboli are more frequent in the posterior circulation and cervical internal carotid artery, in contrast to hemodynamic strokes, which are more common with intracranial internal carotid artery dissection. Intracranial dissection usually affects the internal carotid artery just distal to the cavernous sinus and is often bilateral, none symmetrically (Fig. 8).

The dissecting lesions are subintimal with typical lumen narrowing. Partial or complete repair is seen, sometimes with aneurysm scarring. In a few cases, underlying familial or non-familial arterial wall dysplasias are found. Dissections in children often extend from the classic subintimal location to become subadventitial. Subintimal involvement presents with ischemic strokes (due to occluded perforators, or emboli), whereas a subadventitial extension presents with the development of fusiform aneurysms and subarachnoid hemorrhage.

Moyamoya disease

Moyamoya disease is characterized by progressive stenosis and eventual occlusion of the supraclinoid portion of the internal carotid artery and the adjacent segments of the middle and anterior cerebral arteries. In response, an abnormal vascular network of small collateral vessels develops to bypass the area of occlusion (Fig. 9). It may be idiopathic, related to genetic syndromes (trisomy 21), or acquired damage such as from radiation or sickle cell disease [4]. The disease may affect children who, in turn, tend to present with hemorrhage. In Ganesan's series [22], 26 of the total number of patients

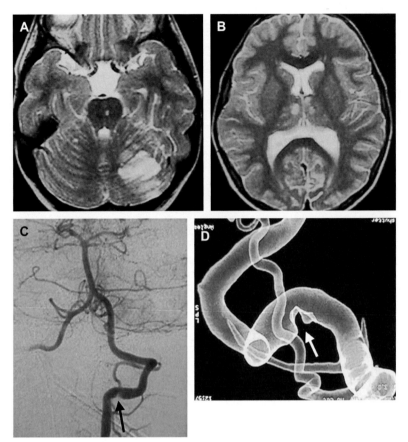

Fig. 7. Six-year-old boy presenting with headaches and vertigo with repeated episodes of vertigo 1 month later. (*A, B*) Axial T2-weighted MR image demonstrates posterior circulation infarcts involving the cerebellum brainstem and thalami. (*C, D*) Angiogram of the left vertebral artery in (*A*) anteroposterior view and (*B*) transparent three-dimensional reconstruction in oblique view demonstrate typical vertebral dissection at the level of C2 (*arrows*). (*From* Berenstein A, Lasjaunias PL, TerBrugge KG, editors. Surgical neuro-angiography, vol. 3. Berlin, Heidelberg, New York: Springer-Verlag; 2006; with permission.)

with AIS had primary or secondary moyamoya disease (14%). In children, multiple transient ischemic attacks and strokes cause cognitive decline and motor impairment [4]. Seizures occur in 33% of children under the age of 6 years. The disorder may remain stable but more often follows a relentlessly progressive course [27,28].

Many pseudo-moyamoya patterns can be seen in childhood with slowly progressive large-vessel vasculopathy and collateralization; however, symmetry, parallel bilateral evolution, transdural angiogenesis, a normal appearance of posterior fossa vascularization, the absence of leptomeningeal collateral circulation with a large transdural contribution, and the role of lenticulo-striate vessels suggest true moyamoya disease.

Hematologic disorders and coagulopathies

Sickle cell disease is the most common hematologic disease associated with AIS. In addition to large-vessel vasculopathy, these children can have small multiple vaso-occlusive strokes, and the nocturnal hypoxemia predicts increased stroke risk [4,29]. The prevalence of cerebrovascular events in patients with sickle cell disease has been reported to be 4.0% and the incidence 0.6 per 100 patient-years. The highest risk for stroke is between the ages of 2 and 5 years. The risk of recurrence is as high as 67% [30,31].

The preventive role of chronic transfusion therapy in sickle cell disease is promising, although certain side effects are being investigated. Transcranial Doppler studies are a noninvasive means of following the progressive large-vessel vasculopathy and determining stroke risk in these patients [32]. The risk associated with angiography in patients with sickle cell disease is decreased with good hydration and transfusion therapy.

The role of prothrombotic disorders is unclear in the pediatric population. Factor V Leiden and

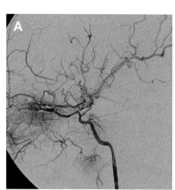
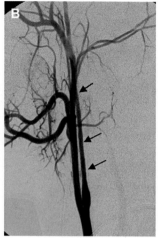
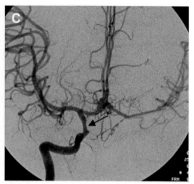

Fig. 8. Six-year-old presenting with transient ischemic symptoms. Angiography shows bilateral spontaneous dissections. (*A*) Lateral view of a left internal carotid angiogram shows complete occlusion of the supraclinoid internal carotid artery. (*B*) Lateral view of a left common carotid angiogram shows narrowing of the entire cervical portion of the internal carotid artery starting just above the carotid bulb (*arrows*). (*C*) Anteroposterior view of an angiogram of the contralateral right internal carotid artery demonstrates a narrowed cavernous and supraclinoid artery (*arrow*). (*From* Berenstein A, Lasjaunias PL, TerBrugge KG, editors. Surgical neuro-angiography, vol. 3. Berlin, Heidelberg, New York: Springer-Verlag; 2006; with permission.)

prothrombin 20210A are probably important in the pathogenesis of AIS, especially in older children [33,34]. Ganesan and colleagues [22] found in a group of AIS patients that only two children had multiple prothrombotic abnormalities (factor V Leiden, homozygous t-MTHFR, and prothrombin 20210 mutation). In the rest of the cases, the abnormalities were transient, and the patients had other risk factors for stroke. The role of hereditary deficiencies of the coagulation inhibitors (protein C, protein S, and antithrombin III) remains debatable, and different case reports and studies have not yet confirmed it. The presence of certain antiphospholipid antibodies, mainly lupus anticoagulant and anticardiolipin antibody, may result in abnormal coagulation and cerebral infarcts in children. Even in the neonatal period, they may be considered a risk factor, being transferred transplacentally from the mother [34]. Acquired deficiencies of protein S, protein C, and the presence of different

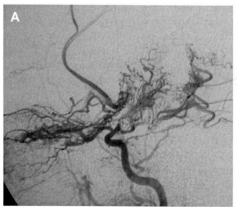
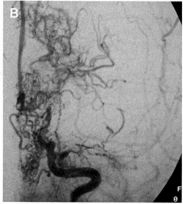

Fig. 9. Cerebral angiograms demonstrate typical appearance of moyamoya disease in a 3-year-old with normal previous development presenting with a hemiplegic episode. (*A,B*) Lateral and anteroposterior views of a left internal carotid artery angiogram demonstrate severe narrowing and near occlusion of the supraclinoid portion of the artery with a classic "puff of smoke" appearance of collaterals. (*From* Berenstein A, Lasjaunias PL, TerBrugge KG, editors. Surgical neuro-angiography, vol. 3. Berlin, Heidelberg, New York: Springer-Verlag; 2006; with permission.)

antibodies have been noted with viral infections and sepsis in patients with stroke, but the importance of these transient deficiencies remains uncertain. Nevertheless, detection of acquired and congenital prothrombotic disorders is essential because of their influence on the initial and long-term treatments.

Metabolic disorders

Homocystinuria due to cystathione beta-synthase deficiency is one of the metabolic disorders known to predispose patients to arterial and venous thrombosis with cerebral infarcts [35,36]. Infarcts may occur before the other features of the disease become evident, such as dislocation of the lens, developmental delay, and a marfanoid habitus [35]. Mitochondrial myopathy, encephalopathy, lactic acidosis, and stroke-like episodes have been described in children with MELAS syndrome. The patients can present with episodes of nausea, vomiting, headaches, seizures, hemiparesis, and cortical blindness. CT and MR imaging typically show areas of infarction but not necessarily in the occipital areas [37].

Migrainous strokes

Although migraine is an accepted cause of cerebral infarction in adults, this association is less well recognized in children. The criteria of the International Headache Society for the diagnosis of migrainous infarction, that is, a history of migrainous neurologic aura and a migrainous crisis identical to the previous one with an incompletely regressive deficit in 7 days, with or without imaging evidence of an infarct of the topography of the symptom presented by the child, are not always fulfilled [38].

PHACE syndrome

PHACE is a rare neurocutaneous syndrome that includes posterior fossa malformations, hemangiomas, arterial anomalies, coarctation of the aorta, cardiac defects, and eye abnormalities. In 1998, Burrows and colleagues [39] reported on eight patients with cervicofacial hemangiomas and cerebrovascular disease. Four of the children had AIS. Other series [40,41] have also demonstrated the susceptibility of the large- and medium-caliber arteries in children with PHACE syndrome. In Burrows' series, the onset of occlusive disease was between birth and 18 months. In Bhattacharya's series, the presentation was much later, that is, from 4 to 14 years of age. The stenotic lesions are mostly located at the anterior division of the internal carotid artery or the M1 segment, as in children with other vascular diseases. Intradural, extracerebral, pial collateral circulation is predominantly recruited. The lesions are usually unilateral and can involve the P1 segment. Treatment includes antiplatelet therapy and surgical cortical stimulation of angiogenesis (Fig. 10).

Hereditary hemorrhagic telangiectasia (Osler-Weber-Rendu Disease)

Hereditary hemorrhage telangiectasia can cause arterial strokes in children. Most of them are embolic in nature and may be septic or aseptic. Usually, they are due to a pulmonary arteriovenous fistula. This

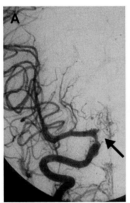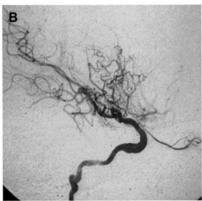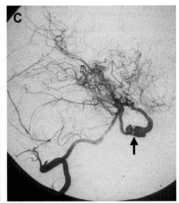

Fig. 10. Six-month-old girl with PHACE syndrome presenting with right-sided fronto-orbital hemangioma, progressive neurologic deficit, chorea, and headaches. (*A, B*) Anteroposterior and lateral views of right internal carotid angiogram demonstrate 50% stenosis of the supraclinoid internal carotid artery and occlusion of the A1 segment of the anterior cerebral artery (*arrow*). (*C*) Lateral view of a vertebral artery angiogram shows occlusion of the distal basilar artery with an extensive network of collateral vessels (*arrow*). Several arterial anomalies are also identified, including segmental agenesis of the right internal carotid artery and a right persisting trigeminal artery. (*From* Berenstein A, Lasjaunias PL, TerBrugge KG, editors. Surgical neuro-angiography, vol. 3. Berlin, Heidelberg, New York: Springer-Verlag; 2006; with permission.)

illness represents a familial type of cerebral stroke disease [42].

Imaging of arterial stroke in children

Advances in neuroimaging modalities have improved the ability to diagnose AIS in children. Imaging studies are helpful in distinguishing ischemic and hemorrhagic infarction from cerebral hemorrhage as a cause of sudden neurologic symptoms. CT is considered to be the modality of choice to detect the presence of hemorrhage acutely after the onset of symptoms, but, as is true in adults, MR imaging has become the first-line neuroimaging modality to confirm the clinical diagnosis of AIS. MR imaging can demonstrate evidence of early infarction even in the first few hours after the onset of symptoms. Diffusion-weighted imaging can demonstrate an acute infarct within minutes from symptom onset. Findings on the apparent diffusion coefficient remain maximally for 4 to 7 days, but in newborns with AIS the apparent diffusion coefficient findings can disappear earlier. MR imaging using diffusion-weighted imaging can sometimes help to estimate the timing of the stroke [4]. Perfusion imaging is another sequence that demonstrates the flow to a certain region of the brain. The penumbra, an area with perfusion abnormality but with no restricted diffusion, is an area of viable brain that is at risk for ischemia. Perfusion and cerebrovascular reactivity studies are important in populations at risk, such as children with sickle cell disease. In these children, perfusion abnormalities or changes in cerebrovascular reactivity may point to an area at risk of stroke before the symptoms appear. In that situation, the patient can be treated with transfusion to prevent the stroke [43].

Vascular investigations are needed to detect arterial disease. Cerebral angiography is still considered the best method to visualize the extra- and intracranial vasculature, but continued improvements and refinements in MR angiography with or with contrast administration have made this modality a realistic noninvasive alternative, particularly in the pediatric population, sparing the child from the harming effects of ionizing radiation. MR angiography is sensitive enough to visualize lesions in the proximal anterior cerebral artery, middle cerebral artery, and distal internal carotid artery (Fig. 11). It can localize the vascular abnormalities as well as make the diagnoses of moyamoya disease and dissections. MR angiography tends to overestimate the length and severity of vessel stenosis. Conventional intra-arterial angiography is still indicated in distal disease and involvement of small arteries [44].

Treatment and management

Treatment recommendations for stroke in children are based on case series, nonrandomized small trials, adult stroke studies, and individual belief and theory. The treatment has been directed toward the underlying pathologic prothrombotic disturbances, supportive care, and neuroprotective agents.

Supportive care that is critical in the prevention of secondary brain injury includes control of blood pressure and volume [45], oxygenation, serum glucose monitoring, and body temperature control. Hyperglycemia is associated with expansion of the stroke [46], and hyperthermia may exacerbate ischemic brain damage. Seizures should be treated promptly. The role of specific therapy for acute stroke in children has not been established. Anticoagulation has been accepted as the treatment of choice in the management of children with cardiogenic thromboembolism, arterial dissections, and prothrombotic disorders. Antiplatelet medications are used more in the vasculopathies, in idiopathic strokes, and as secondary prevention of AIS. The role of systemic intravenous or intra-arterial thrombolytic therapy, currently actively pursued in adults, has rarely been explored in children with acute onset of AIS. The differences in stroke mechanisms, the coagulation system function, the limited access to patients in time for thrombolysis, and the measures of acute stroke severity are all barriers for thrombolytic treatment in children's stroke [47].

Treatment in neck dissections with emboli includes neck immobilization with sand bags or a collar and anticoagulants (low molecular weight heparin at the acute stage, followed by warfarin or low molecular weight heparin for 3 to 6 months).

Lately, two separate, evidence-based treatment guidelines have been published—the *Chest* and the United Kingdom guidelines. Both trials are focusing on AIS in children beyond the newborn period and were created by panels of pediatric neurologists and hematologists [48–50].

Outcome and prognosis

The prognosis for children after stroke has generally been thought to be better than that for adults, although few reports in the literature present sufficient data regarding long-term follow-up to substantiate this observation. In addition, because of the fact that pediatric arterial stroke is multifactorial (as opposed to that in adults), one must realize that the outcome data published in the literature often ignore the various etiologies responsible for pediatric ischemia and combine the data by age groups rather then by etiology.

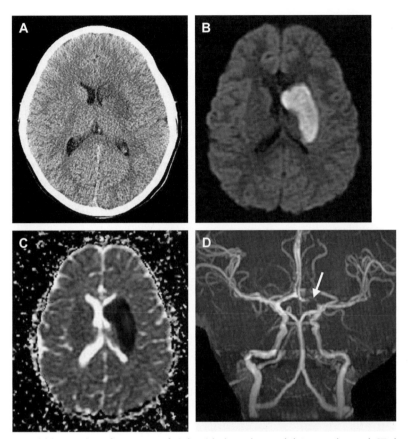

Fig. 11. Seven-year-old boy 1 day after onset of right-sided weakness. (*A*) Non-enhanced CT demonstrates an infarct in the basal ganglia including the head of caudate and anterior limb of the internal capsule. (*B, C*) Diffusion-weighted MR image and apparent diffusion coefficient map demonstrate an acute stroke with restricted diffusion. (*D*) MR angiography demonstrates a filling defect and occlusion of the A1 segment of the left anterior cerebral artery (*arrow*) as well as irregularity in the M1 segment of the middle cerebral artery. The area of vessel occlusion and the distribution of infarct are compatible with an occlusion of the recurrent artery of hubner.

Among a prospectively collected series of 123 Canadian children (33 neonates, 90 infants and children) presenting with arterial stroke, it was demonstrated that the neonates with arterial ischemia had better primary outcomes than the older infants and children (60% good outcome versus 48% in older children). In the same cohort, among the children with AIS, 67% did not recover according to parental response on follow-up [51]. In another study of 31 children with AIS, the fatality rate was 13% in the first 6 months after the event, and 29% of the children had severe disability. That study showed that an altered level of consciousness, seizures, or both were related to death and poor outcome. A large cortical stroke in comparison with a subcortical stroke was also shown to be a risk factor for poor outcome [52]. Schoenberg and colleagues [1] reported that although 84% of children survived 5 years after the onset of stroke, residual deficits were found in 75% of the surviving

patients. Similarly, long-term follow-up of children after neonatal ischemic stroke has revealed mental and motor developmental delay in nearly all patients [53]; therefore, it seems that the outcome in childhood stroke is not as good as previously thought.

The risk of recurrent stroke in children ranges from 10% to 25% in treated patients to as high as 50% in untreated children [47]. Recurrence is maximal in the first 6 months and increases in the presence of vasculopathy and other risk factors [47,54]. Certain disorders such as sickle cell disease are known to be associated with a high rate of recurrence [55].

Childhood stroke is a multifactorial disease different from that in adults that usually causes significant long-term morbidity. It is hoped that the change in the approach to childhood stroke, the evolution in treatment, and the major advances in the imaging of stroke and diagnosis of risk factors will contribute to improved treatment in the acute phase and prevention of a recurrent event.

References

[1] Schoenberg BS, Mellinger JF, Schoenberg DG. Cerebrovascular disease in infants and children: a study of incidence, clinical features, and survival. Neurology 1978;28(8):763–8.

[2] Broderick J, Talbot GT, Prenger E, et al. Stroke in children within a major metropolitan area: the surprising importance of intracerebral hemorrhage. J Child Neurol 1993;8:250–5.

[3] Giroud M, Lemesle M, Gouyon JB, et al. Cerebrovascular disease in children under 16 years of age in the city of Dijon, Franc: a study of incidence and clinical features from 1983 to 1993. J Clin Epidemiol 1995;48(11):1343–8.

[4] deVeber G. Stroke and the child's brain: an overview of epidemiology, syndromes and risk factors. Curr Opin Neurol 2002;15(2):133–8.

[5] Kuhle S, Mitchell L, Andrew M, et al. Urgent clinical challenges in children with ischemic stroke: analysis of 1065 patients from the 1-800-NO-CLOTS pediatric stroke telephone consultation service. Stroke 2006;37:116–22.

[6] Bouza H, Rutherford M, Acolet D, et al. Evolution of early hemiplegic signs in full-term infants with unilateral brain lesions in the neonatal period: a prospective study. Neuropediatrics 1994; 25(4):201–7.

[7] Golomb MR, MacGregor DL, Domi T, et al. Presumed pre- or perinatal arterial ischemic stroke: risk factors and outcomes. Ann Neurol 2001;50: 163–8.

[8] Lanska MJ, Lanska DJ, Horwitz SJ, et al. Presentation, clinical course, and outcome of childhood stroke. Pediatr Neurol 1991;7(5):333–41.

[9] Aydinli N, Tatli B, Çaliskan M, et al. Stroke in childhood: experience in Istanbul, Turkey. J Trop Pediatr 2006;52(3):158–62.

[10] Miller G, Mamourian AC, Tesman JR, et al. Long-term MRI changes in brain after pediatric open heart surgery. J Child Neurol 1994;9(4):390–7.

[11] Kaplan DM, McCrindle B, deVeber GA. Stroke and congenital heart disease: frequency and predictors of stroke associated with cardiac catheterization and surgery in infants and children. Neurology 1999;52(6 Suppl 2):A151.

[12] Majersik JJ, Skalabrin EJ. Single-gene stroke disorders. Semin Neurol 2006;26(1):33–48.

[13] Gallitelli M, Pasculli G, Fiore T, et al. Emergencies in hereditary haemorrhagic telangiectasia. QJM 2006;99(1):15–22.

[14] Chiu CH, Lin TY, Huang YC. Cranial nerve palsies and cerebral infarction in a young infant with meningococcal meningitis. Scand J Infect Dis 1995;27(1):75–6.

[15] Askalan R, Laughlin S, Supriya M, et al. Chickenpox and stroke in childhood: a study of frequency and causation. Stroke 2001;32:1257–62.

[16] Moriarty DM, Haller JO, Loh JP, et al. Cerebral infarction in pediatric acquired immunodeficiency syndrome. Pediatr Radiol 1994;24(8): 611–2.

[17] Chabrier S, Rodesch G, Lasjaunias P, et al. Transient cerebral arteriopathy: a disorder recognized by serial angiograms in children with stroke. J Child Neurol 1998;13(1):27–32.

[18] Syrjanen J. Infection as a risk factor for cerebral infarction. Eur Heart J 1993;14(Suppl K):17–9.

[19] Berger TM, Caduff JH, Gebbers JO. Fatal varicella-zoster virus antigen-positive giant cell arteritis of the central nervous system. Pediatr Infect Dis J 2000;19(7):653–6.

[20] Lanthier S, Lortie A, Michaud J, et al. Isolated angiitis of the CNS in children. Neurology 2001; 56(7):834–42.

[21] Kohrman MH, Huttenlocher PR. Takayasu arteritis: a treatable cause of stroke in infancy. Pediatr Neurol 1986;2(3):154–8.

[22] Ganesan V, Prengler M, McShane MA, et al. Investigation of risk factors in children with arterial ischemic stroke. Ann Neurol 2003;53: 167–73.

[23] Chabrier S, Lasjaunias P, Husson B, et al. Ischemic stroke from dissection of the craniocervical arteries in childhood: report of 12 patients. Eur J Paediatr Neurol 2003;7(1):39–42.

[24] Schievink WI, Mokri B, Piepgras DG. Spontaneous dissections of cervicocephalic arteries in childhood and adolescence. Neurology 1994;44(9): 1607–12.

[25] Fullerton HJ, Johnston SC, Smith WS. Arterial dissection and stroke in children. Neurology 2001;57(7):1155–60.

[26] Rafay MF, Armstrong D, Deveber G, et al. Craniocervical arterial dissection in children: clinical and radiographic presentation and outcome. J Child Neurol 2006;21(1):8–16.

[27] Maki Y, Enomoto T. Moyamoya disease. Childs Nerv Syst 1988;4(4):204–12.

[28] Yoshida S, Matsumoto S, Ban S, et al. Moyamoya disease progressing from unilateral to bilateral involvement–case report. Neurol Med Chir (Tokyo) 1992;32(12):900–3.

[29] Kirkham FJ, Hewes DK, Prengler M, et al. Nocturnal hypoxemia and central nervous system events in sickle cell disease. Lancet 2001;357:1656–9.

[30] Prengler M, Pavlakis SG, Prohovnik I, et al. Sickle cell disease: the neurological complications. Ann Neurol 2002;51:543–52.

[31] Ohene-Frempong K, Weiner SJ, Sleeper LA, et al. Cerebrovascular accidents in sickle cell disease: rates and risk factors. Blood 1998;91(1):288–94.

[32] Lee MT, Piomelli S, Granger S, et al. Stroke prevention trial in sickle cell anemia (STOP): extended follow-up and final results. Blood 2006;108(3):847–52.

[33] Kenet G, Sadetzki S, Murad H, et al. Factor V Leiden and antiphospholipid antibodies are significant risk factors for ischemic stroke in children. Stroke 2000;31:1283–8.

[34] Nowak-Göttl U, Sträter R, Junker R, et al. Lipoprotein (a) and genetic polymorphisms of clotting factor V, prothrombin, and methylenetetrahydrofolate reductase are risk factors of spontaneous ischemic stroke in childhood. Blood 1999;94:3678–82.

[35] van Beynum IM, Smeitink JA, den Heijer M, et al. Hyperhomocysteinemia: a risk factor for ischemic stroke in children. Circulation 1999;99:2070–2.

[36] Mudd SH, Skovby F, Levy HL, et al. The natural history of homocystinuria due to cystathionine beta-synthase deficiency. Am J Hum Genet 1985;37(1):1–31.

[37] Riikonen R, Santavuori P. Hereditary and acquired risk factors for childhood stroke. Neuropediatrics 1994;25(5):227–33.

[38] Ebinger F, Boor R, Gawehn J, et al. Ischemic stroke and migraine in childhood: coincidence or causal relation? J Child Neurol 1999;14(7):451–5.

[39] Burrows PE, Robertson RL, Mulliken JB, et al. Cerebral vasculopathy and neurologic sequelae in infants with cervicofacial hemangioma: report of eight patients. Radiology 1998;207:601–7.

[40] Bhattacharya JJ, Luo CB, Alvarez H, et al. PHACES syndrome: a review of eight previously unreported cases with late arterial occlusions. Neuroradiology 2004;46(3):227–33.

[41] Drolet BA, Dohil M, Golomb MR, et al. Early stroke and cerebral vasculopathy in children with facial hemangiomas and PHACE association. Pediatrics 2006;117:959–64.

[42] Kjeldsen AD, Oxhoj H, Andersen PE, et al. Prevalence of pulmonary arteriovenous malformations (PAVMs) and occurrence of neurological symptoms in patients with hereditary haemorrhagic telangiectasia (HHT). J Intern Med 2000;248(3):255–62.

[43] Gadian DG, Calamante F, Kirkham FJ, et al. Diffusion and perfusion magnetic resonance imaging in childhood stroke. J Child Neurol 2000;15:279–83.

[44] Husson B, Lasjaunias P. Radiological approach to disorders of arterial brain vessels associated with childhood arterial stroke–a comparison between MRA and contrast angiography. Pediatr Radiol 2004;34:10–5.

[45] Trescher WH. Ischemic stroke syndromes in childhood. Pediatr Ann 1992;21(6):374–83.

[46] Baird TA, Parsons MW, Phanh T, et al. Persistent poststroke hyperglycemia is independently associated with infarct expansion and worse clinical outcome. Stroke 2003;34:2208–14.

[47] Kirton A, deVeber G. Therapeutic approaches and advances in pediatric stroke. NeuroRx 2006;3:133–42.

[48] Monagle P, Chan A, Massicotte P, et al. Antithrombotic therapy in children: the Seventh ACCP Conference on Antithrombotic and Thrombolytic Therapy. Chest 2004;126:645S–87S.

[49] Paediatric Stroke Working Group. Stroke in childhood: clinical guidelines for diagnosis, management and rehabilitation. 2004. Available at: http://www.rcplondon.ac.uk/pubs/books/childstroke/. Accessed June 1, 2005.

[50] deVeber G. In pursuit of evidence-based treatments for paediatric stroke: the UK and Chest guidelines. Lancet Neurol 2005;4:432–6.

[51] deVeber G, MacGregor D, Curtis R, et al. Neurologic outcome in survivors of childhood arterial ischemic stroke and sinovenous thrombosis. J Child Neurol 2000;15:316–24.

[52] Delsing BJ, Castmen-Berrevoets CE, Appel IM. Early prognostic indicator of outcome in ischemic childhood stroke. Pediatr Neurol 2001;24:283–9.

[53] Koelfen W, Freund M, Konig S, et al. Results of parenchymal and angiographic magnetic resonance imaging and neuropsychological testing of children after stroke as neonates. Eur J Pediatr 1993;152:1030–5.

[54] Strater R, Becker S, von Eckardstein A, et al. Prospective assessment of risk factors for recurrent stroke during childhood: a 5-year follow-up study. Lancet 2002;360:1540–5.

[55] Pegelow CH, Adams RJ, McKie V, et al. Risk of recurrent stroke in patients with sickle cell disease treated with erythrocyte transfusions. J Pediatr 1995;126(6):896–9.

ELSEVIER
SAUNDERS

NEUROIMAGING
CLINICS
OF NORTH AMERICA

Neuroimag Clin N Am 17 (2007) 189–206

Vein of Galen Aneurysmal Malformations

H. Alvarez, MD, R. Garcia Monaco, MD, G. Rodesch, MD, PhD,
M. Sachet, MD, T. Krings, MD, PhD, Pierre Lasjaunias, MD, PhD*

The first description of a possible vein of Galen aneurysmal malformation (VGAM) was reported in 1895 by Steinheil (cited by Dandy [1] in 1928), but that lesion was, in fact, a cerebral arteriovenous malformation (AVM) of the diencephalon draining into a dilated vein of Galen. The first attempts to treat a VGAM were recorded at the beginning of the last century and described an infant who presented with intracranial hypertension and subsequently underwent bilateral internal carotid artery ligations. In 1946, Jeager reported bilateral arteriovenous communications draining into a dilated vein of Galen, while Boldrey and Miller [2] in 1949 treated two similar patients with arterial ligations. Only the last case seems to correspond to a true VGAM. Litvak [3] in 1960, Raimondi [4] in 1972, Clarisse [5] in 1978, and Diebler [6] in 1981 suggested the possible existence of true and false VGAMs.

More recently, anatomic and embryologic [7] evidence has allowed us to categorize a VGAM as a specific choroidal malformation that is different from a cerebral AVM draining into a dilated but not malformed vein of Galen. Several investigators [8–10] have established the relationship between VGAM and heart failure in neonates. In 1964 in a review of 34 patients, Gold [11] described the following three consecutive clinical stages in patients with VGAMs: (1) neonates with cardiac insufficiency, (2) infants and young children with hydrocephalus and seizures, and (3) older children or adults with headaches and subarachnoid hemorrhage. In 1978, Amacher [12] added a fourth group that included neonates and infants with macrocephaly and minimal cardiac symptoms. In an excellent review, Johnston and colleagues [13] analyzed in an exhaustive fashion the clinical presentations of VGAMs. In 82 infants, he found the following symptoms: cerebrospinal fluid (CSF) disorders (70%), neurologic deficits (31%), and neurocognitive delay (12%). Among children aged 1 to 5 years, these symptoms occurred in 61%, 33%, and 5%, respectively. These clinical groups do not match those encountered by the authors in their practice. This difference may be due to the inclusion of VGAMs and cerebral AVMs

Service de Neuroradiologie Diagnostique et Thérapeutique, Hôpital Bicêtre 78, rue du Général Leclerc, 94275 Le Kremlin-Bicêtre, Paris, France
* Corresponding author.
E-mail address: pierre.lasjaunias@bct.aphp.fr (P. Lasjaunias).

doi:10.1016/j.nic.2007.02.005

in the previous analysis and the fact that the therapeutic approach did not take into account the window of opportunity for treatment of VGAMs.

Between October 1984 and 2002, 317 children less than 16 years of age with VGAMs were studied at the authors' center. Of this cohort, 233 patients were treated with endovascular embolization (216 at the authors' hospital). Of the 216 patients, 23 died despite being treated with embolization or due to procedure-related complications (10.6%). Twenty of the 193 surviving patients were severely retarded (10.4%), 30 were moderately retarded (15.6%), and 143 (74%) were neurologically normal on follow-up. Management of these patients has required the involvement of anesthesia, neurology, and pediatric neurosurgery teams at the authors' center for the last 20 years. The contributions to the management of VGAM offered by the authors' approach include the ability to identify the specific type of lesion, to anticipate the natural clinical course of the disease, and to institute treatment within the window of opportunity. The observations detailed in this review are derived from the authors' experience [14,15].

Classification

Vein of galen aneurysmal malformation

A VGAM is a choroidal type of AVM. The lesion is supplied by the choroidal arteries. The choroidal shunt drains into a dilated vein, which Raybaud and colleagues [7] first recognized as an ectatic vein, which is the median vein of the prosencephalon, the embryonic precursor of the vein of Galen. This embryonic vein drains only the choroidal system and does not connect with the deep venous system. It does not become the vein of Galen until

communications with the thalamostriate and internal cerebral veins develop. In patients with VGAMs, these latter communications do not form, and the thalamostriate veins drain into the posterior and inferior thalamic (diencephalic) veins and secondarily join the anterior confluence, a subtemporal vein, or (more often) the lateral mesencephalic vein to open into the superior petrosal sinuses, which demonstrate a typical epsilon shape ("epsilon vein") on the lateral angiogram (Fig. 1) [14,15]. Persistence of this venous arrangement is identical to that seen early in life before the 12th week of gestation. This pattern allows one to establish the time at which the malformation developed, and one may consider a VGAM to be the result of an error in the early phase of vasculogenesis. Prenatal diagnosis of VGAM may be made as early as the second trimester of intrauterine life by sonography or MR imaging. In the authors' series of patients, 29.3% of cases were diagnosed in utero.

Vein of galen aneurysmal dilatation

Vein of Galen aneurysmal dilatations correspond to AVMs localized in the subpial space, either supra- or infratentorially, which drain into one of the usual tributaries of the vein of Galen and result in its overload and dilatation. This dilatation of the vein of Galen is variable and depends on the outflow obstruction due to stenoses or thrombosis where the vein joins the straight sinus. In this type of lesion, the vein of Galen is fully developed and drains not only the lesion but also the adjacent brain parenchyma. The arteriovenous shunts are located in the cerebellum, brainstem, or in the deep supratentorial territories that normally drain into the vein of Galen. Some tectal AVMs (supplied by transcerebral arteries) may mimic true choroidal VGAMs. Careful

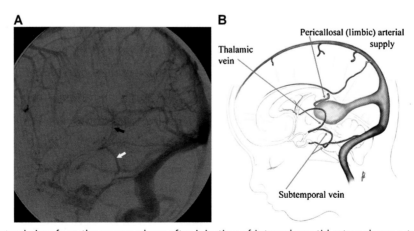

Fig. 1. (A) Lateral view from the venous phase after injection of internal carotid artery shows a typical venous epsilon shape formed by thalamic (*black arrow*) and lateral perimesencephalic (*white arrow*) veins without drainage through the vein of Galen, straight, or falcine sinus. (B) Diagram illustrating the same configuration.

analysis of the arterial vascularization of lesions (always choroidal or subependymal in VGAMs) and of venous drainage (absence of connections with deep veins in VGAMs) allows one to arrive at the correct diagnosis. The prenatal diagnosis of a vein of Galen dilatation is uncommon, and the frequency of this lesion in neonates and infants is low. Clinical manifestations of vein of Galen dilatation include neurologic deficits, intracranial hemorrhages, or, in the very young, subsequent delayed psychomotor development. Epilepsy is not common owing to the deep localization of the lesions, and heart failure is also uncommon because these lesions are found in older children.

Vein of galen varix

This lesion refers to a varicose dilatation of the vein of Galen without an underlying arteriovenous shunt and drains normal brain parenchyma (Fig. 2). Two types of vein of Galen varices are encountered in children. The first is a transient dilatation of the vein of Galen in neonates presenting with cardiac failure of a different origin. This venous dilatation persists for a few days postnatally and then disappears on follow-up ultrasound studies. The dilatation does not lead to any symptoms, and its disappearance parallels cardiovascular improvement. The second type of vein of Galen varix is associated with complex developmental venous anomalies draining an entire hemisphere into the deep venous system. This subtype of varix does not result in any specific symptoms, but, over time, some patients may show symptoms of venous ischemia due to insufficient venous drainage.

Dural vein of galen dilatation

These malformations belong to a group of acquired dural lesions that develop in the wall of the vein of Galen or at the venous-sinus junction [16,17]. In nearly all patients, the straight sinus is thrombosed. These lesions occur almost exclusively in adults. In children, similar dural arteriovenous shunts develop secondarily to a complete thrombosis of the vein of Galen or of the falcine sinus. This thrombosis stimulates angiogenesis. At this level, angiogenesis is favored by pre-existing vasa vasorum in the vein of Galen wall.

Vein of galen aneurysmal malformation

Architecture and pathophysiology

The arterial supply of a VGAM usually involves all of the choroidal arteries, including anterior choroidal contributions (Fig. 3). It may also receive significant contributions from the subependymal network (Fig. 4) originating from the posterior circle of Willis. These arteries should be differentiated from transmesencephalic ones, because the involvement of the latter excludes the diagnosis of VGAM and indicates a tectal and not a choroidal AVM. The subependymal arteries pierce the floor of the third ventricle and run under the ependyma to join the choroid fissure, where they contribute to the blood supply of the lesion. Subependymal and thalamo-perforating contributions supply the shunt as accessories that are recruited by the sump effect of the venous drainage, and they usually disappear following proper occlusion of the most prominent shunts. Cerebellar arteries do not supply a VGAM except indirectly through their dural branches, which can be enlarged because they may participate in the supply to the vasa vasorum at the veno-dural junction. A persistent limbic arterial arch, which bridges the cortical branches of the anterior choroidal artery initially (Fig. 5) and the posterior cerebral artery, is seen in nearly one half of neonatal VGAM cases. This limbic arch should be distinguished from subcallosal and subforniceal

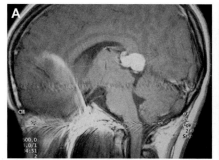 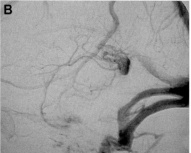

Fig. 2. Vein of Galen aneurysmal dilatation without shunt. (*A*) Midsagittal post contrast T1-weighted MR image in a 14-year-old child who presented with meningitis. A dilatation of the vein of Galen was incidentally discovered. The vein is bright due to slow blood flow. (*B*) Venous phase of angiogram, lateral view after injection of internal carotid artery confirms dilated vein of Galen that receives blood from the internal cerebral and atrial veins. There is no evidence of an arteriovenous shunt.

A   **B**

Fig. 3. (A) Internal carotid injection in lateral view showing arterial vascularization of the vein of Galen malformation through the anterior (*black arrow*) and posterior (*arrowhead*) choroidal systems and by subcallosal and subforniceal vessels arising from the anterior cerebral artery (*wavy arrow*). Note the anterior opening of shunts into a choroidal collector vein (*white arrow*). (B) Schematic representation of the same vascular arrangement.

supply to the choroidal shunts. The arch regresses (matures) after obliteration of the VGAM by means of embolization.

The nidus of a VGAM is usually located in the midline and receives bilateral supply. Generally, two types of angioarchitecture are encountered: choroidal and mural (see Fig. 4). The former corresponds to a primitive condition involving all of the choroidal arteries and an interposed network before opening into the large venous pouch. This condition is encountered in most neonates with severe symptoms. The latter type corresponds to direct arteriovenous fistulas within the wall of the median vein of the prosencephalon. The fistulas may be single or, more often, multiple and converge into a single venous chamber or into multiple venous

chambers located along the anterior aspect of a venous pouch or along one dilated choroidal vein before reaching the venous pouch. The mural form is better tolerated clinically than the choroidal form. Mixed forms may occur, such as those with a choroidal nidus and high-flow fistulas located in the wall of the venous pouch.

The venous drainage of the choroidal shunt is always via a median prosencephalic vein and has no communication with the deep venous system. The choroidal veins are the embryonic tributaries of the median vein, and, potentially, the choroidal nidus may drain into the choroidal veins before they join the median pontomesencephalic vein. The connection between the medial pontomesencephalic vein and the choroidal veins may result in

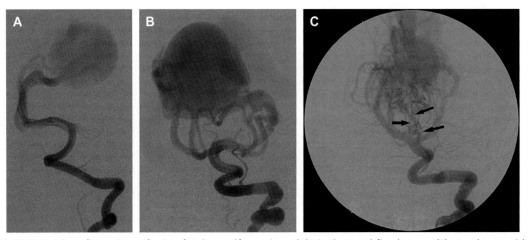

Fig. 4. Arterial configurations of vein of Galen malformations. (A) Single mural fistula type. (B) Mural type with multiple fistulas fed by the posterior choroidal arteries. (C) Choroidal type with vascular nidus fed by choroidal and subependymal (*arrows*) arteries originating from the P1 segments of both posterior cerebral arteries.

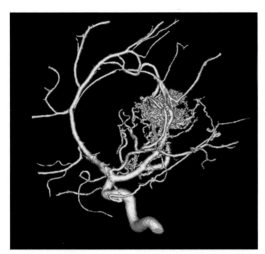

Fig. 5. Three-dimensional reformation of an internal carotid artery injection in a lateral and slightly anterior oblique projection shows persistence of the limbic arch.

reflux into the pial venous system due to communications between the choroidal and striate veins (Fig. 6). This arrangement is found in untreated older children with advanced VGAMs or in those who have undergone occlusion of their venous drainage without complete embolization of the arterial components. A connection with the choroidal veins must be sought out by angiography; their visualization is a contraindication to embolization by the venous route. Intraventricular bleeds and cerebral venous infarctions may occur after complete occlusion of a VGAM via the venous route if the lesion drained into the choroidal, subependymal, or striate venous systems. Reflux into the pial venous system leads to risks of seizures and bleeds similar to those associated with brain AVMs, which need urgent treatment, and alters the standard algorithm of management for VGAMs.

Dilatation of the median pontomesencephalic vein is variable and not related to the architecture of a choroidal or mural VGAM. This vein opens most commonly into a large falcine sinus; stenoses at the veno-sinus junction are occasionally encountered. These stenoses may increase the cerebral venous pressure, but, conversely, they improve heart function by decreasing overload.

The VGAM drains into the straight sinus and uses the posterior sinuses as a route of drainage. This implies that the deep cerebral venous system is

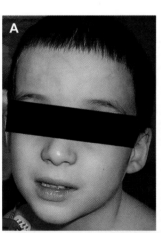

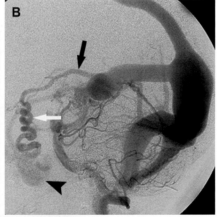

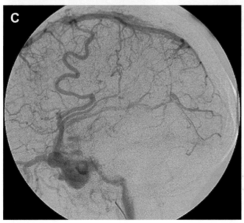

Fig. 6. (A) Photograph of a 6-year-old child with a choroidal type of vein of Galen malformation diagnosed 1 year previously when he presented with macrocrania, facial vein prominence, but no neurocognitive symptoms. (B) Lateral angiographic view from injection of a vertebral artery shows subependymal (black arrow) and inferior striate (white arrow) reflux that secondarily drained into the cavernous sinus (arrowhead). (C) Venous phase of internal carotid artery injection in lateral view showing the opening of the cerebral venous drainage in the cavernous sinus, which also receives the pial reflux of the malformation. Urgent embolization was indicated in this case.

drained by alternative pathways. As mentioned previously, an alternate route of drainage is via thalamic and subtemporal or lateromesencephalic veins, demonstrating typical epsilon shapes on the lateral angiogram [14,15]. Visualization of the epsilon vein following contrast injection into the internal carotid arteries is a favorable sign and predicts a good neurologic prognosis.

The cavernous sinuses are another alternative route of venous cerebral drainage in patients who have a VGAM. During the prenatal period and the first months of life, the cavernous sinuses do not connect with the cerebral veins. At a later time, the cavernous sinuses mature and become able to "capture" blood from the sylvian veins, offering the brain a potential drainage pathway through the orbits, pterygoid plexuses, or inferior petrosal sinuses (Fig. 7). Cerebral venous drainage via the ophthalmic veins increases the clinical visibility of the facial and scalp veins (see Fig 6). Dilatation of the facial veins in infants is an indication that cerebral venous drainage is occurring via the cavernous sinuses and is associated with a good prognosis. Rarely, facial venous congestion may result in nasal mucosal swelling and mild epistaxis.

Maturation of the jugular bulbs and of the venous sinuses at the base of the skull occurs during the peri- and postnatal periods. This process of maturation encompasses remodeling of the torcular, regression of the embryonic occipital and marginal sinuses, and definite formation of the jugular bulbs [18]. These maturation processes may be disturbed by the presence of high-flow shunts or by macrocephaly, which alters the normal development of the skull base. Processes that interfere with venous maturation at the base of the skull are also seen with high-flow pial arteriovenous fistulas in newborns and infants.

The prognosis for infants who have a VGAM depends largely on the evolution of the maturation of both sino-jugular junctions. Partial restriction of venous outflow into a jugular bulb together with drainage into the cavernous sinuses allows for normal cerebral venous drainage through the ophthalmic veins or the veins of the foramen ovale. If the stenosis of a jugular bulb is more pronounced, or if the jugular bulb is thrombosed, the VGAM and the brain use the cavernous sinuses to drain (see Fig. 6), leading to cerebral venous hypertension. This situation may be further aggravated in patients with bilateral sigmoid sinus thrombosis (Fig. 8) Cerebral venous drainage via the cavernous sinuses may be uni- or bilateral. In some patients, bi-hemispheric drainage is accomplished via the sylvian veins draining into only one cavernous sinus. If this occurs, unilateral exophthalmos may develop if the venous drainage recruits the ophthalmic systems. Similarly, epistaxis may develop owing to engorgement of the nasal mucosa and the facial veins. Obstructed venous drainage, particularly a lack of recruitment of the cavernous sinuses, may lead to a "pseudophlebitic" appearance of the cortical veins on angiography (Fig. 9). The combination of jugular bulb occlusion and venous pial reflux may exist for a few years, and some children with undiagnosed VGAM may present late with intracerebral hematomas or subdural or subarachnoid hemorrhage.

The infratentorial consequence of sinus occlusion is cerebral tonsillar herniation [19]. Tonsillar herniation is secondary to cerebellar pial congestion and is only seen in its presence. It may disappear with correction of the arteriovenous shunts provided that the herniation has not existed for a long time (Fig. 10).

Another fundamental aspect of neonatal and infant anatomy and CSF physiology is that the

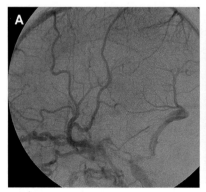
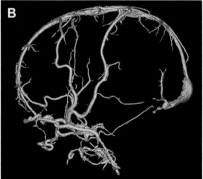

Fig. 7. Venous architecture. (*A*) Venous phase from injection of an internal carotid artery (lateral view) shows drainage being captured by a cavernous sinus in a 9-month-old child. Secondaryly, the flow is opening into the ophthalmic veins and inferior petrosal sinus. (*B*) Same image in a three-dimensional reformation.

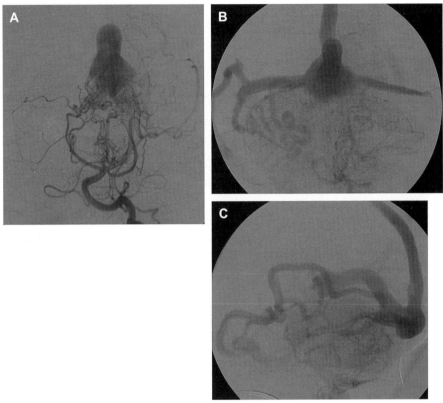

Fig. 8. Findings in a 3.5-year-old child with macrocrania since the age of 2 months and diagnosed with a vein of Galen malformation at 15 months of age. Because of mismanagement, treatment was started at 30 months age. (*A*) Arterial phase from a vertebral artery injection (frontal view) at age 4 years shows persistent flow in the malformation. (*B*, *C*) Venous phase (*B* is frontal and *C* is lateral) shows evolution to progressive bilateral thrombosis of the sigmoid sinuses and subsequent development of pial reflux through the temporal veins as well as into the deep subependymal veins. The child sustained uncontrollable seizures. Emergent occlusion of the malformation via an arterial route was indicated.

pacchionian granulations are not functional during the first months of life; therefore, CSF must be absorbed, at least partly, via the medullary veins [19,20]. The association of this immaturity of the pacchionian granulations and venous hypertension arising from stenoses at the skull base results in an unbalanced hydrovenous state, leading eventually to hydrocephalus. Mechanical compression of the

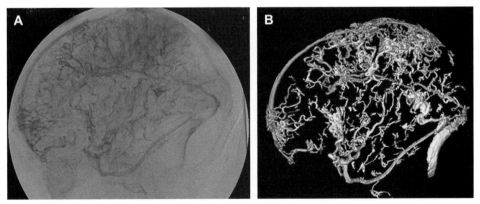

Fig. 9. (*A*) Lateral view from an internal carotid artery injection shows pseudophlebitic aspect of the cortical veins due to their congestion by occlusion of the sigmoid sinus associated with insufficient cavernous sinus "capture" of venous blood. (*B*) Corresponding three-dimensional reformation shows the same appearance of the venous collateral circulation.

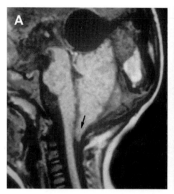
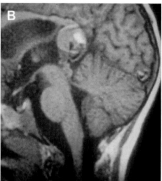
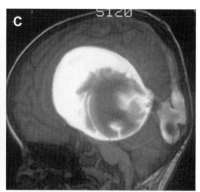

Fig. 10. (*A*) MR imaging before embolization shows a vein of Galen malformation and cerebral tonsillar herniation (*arrow*). (*B*) After embolization, MR imaging in the same patient shows occlusion of the vascular malformation and resolution of the tonsillar herniation. (*C*) MR imaging in a different child shows a voluminous vein of Galen malformation without tonsillar herniation. These cases illustrate the hydrodynamic disturbance nature of tonsillar herniation in the vein of Galen malformation rather than a mechanical one.

mesencephalic aqueduct should not be considered to be the primary cause of the hydrodynamic disorders at this age in VGAM patients; in reality, the aqueduct is patent in almost patients [6,20].

Untreated VGAMs evolve toward chronic venous ischemia manifested by the development of subcortical white matter calcifications and subependymal atrophy with ventricular dilatation (Fig. 11). These calcifications reflect deep hydrovenous watershed failure, and they occur when the compliance of the medullary veins loses its normal ventricular-cortical gradient. These calcifications are usually bilateral and symmetrical, but they may be asymmetrical and mostly unilateral in shunted children (often on the side opposite to the shunt). Subependymal atrophy is primarily seen in the occipital regions. It may be dramatic, and it seems to be at least partially related to an abnormal postnatal development of the corpus callosum. Spontaneous thromboses of isolated cortical veins are also possible in untreated patients with VGAM.

Clinical manifestations

Clinical manifestations of patients who have VGAMs are mainly divided into those related to high output cardiac failure and those involving neurologic symptoms due to venous congestion and abnormal CSF flow. Their severity and tolerability are variable and are related to the angioarchitecture of the VGAM and the age of the child.

Cardiac manifestations

The cerebral arteriovenous shunts result in a larger volume of venous return to the right side of the

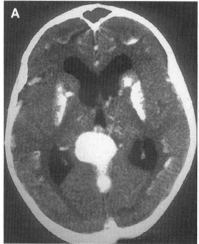
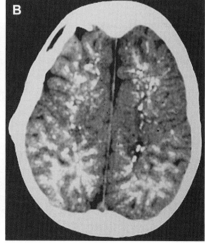

Fig. 11. (*A, B*) Axial CT studies showing subependymal and cortical calcifications as a result of chronic venous ischemia in a vein of Galen malformation.

heart and lead to dilatation of the right-sided chambers [21]. At the same time, there is increased pulmonary blood flow and resultant pulmonary hypertension. All of this leads to failure of the left chambers (due to increased preload). Prenatal development of congestive heart failure is sonographically diagnosed by supraventricular extrasystole, tricuspid valve insufficiency, and tachycardia (over 200 beats per minute) and portrays a poor prognosis. In its most severe form, it may be associated with multiorgan failure and irreversible brain damage ("melting" brain). Termination of pregnancy should be considered in this scenario (performed in 3 of 93 of fetuses in the authors' series). In the authors' experience, 22% of children with a prenatal diagnosis have irreversible cerebral damage at birth and die soon thereafter. The remaining infants should undergo embolization at a time dependent on their individual response to medical cardiac treatment. Antenatal diagnosis is not an indication to perform early delivery, interruption of pregnancy, or cesarian section at term [22].

In the neonatal period, cardiac symptoms vary from mild overload to cardiogenic shock [21–24]. In the mildest form, only cardiomegaly is present. During the neonatal period, there is a brief time (approximately the first 3 days of life) of clinical stabilization, but, shortly afterward, congestive heart failure worsens, then stabilizes, and finally improves with appropriate medical management. At birth, the transition between fetal and adult circulations imposes great demands on the myocardium, which already has a limited function because it contains a relatively high proportion of noncontractile fibers that, in combination with the relative immaturity of the sympathetic nervous system, explain the worsening of heart function during the first week of life. Symptoms depend on the volume of the cerebral arteriovenous shunts but, for the most part, are a reflection of the state of maturation of the cardiopulmonary system. Mild symptoms include feeding difficulties, lack of weight gain, and tachycardia. Chest radiographs show cardiomegaly, especially involving the right side. If the cardiac failure is mild, medical treatment generally suffices. Diuretics are initiated to reduce cardiac preload. One of the most important goals of medical treatment is to permit normal oral feeding, which ensures weight gain and allows the child to go home and to return at 5 months of age for embolization.

Not uncommonly, infections may lead to decompensation of the cardiac status, necessitating immediate treatment of the VGAM. Echocardiography is the best method to evaluate the cardiac consequences of the VGAM. In patients with severe heart failure, mechanical ventilation is needed a few hours after birth. This ventilation reduces oxygen needs and improves myocardial performance. Adjustments in the inspired fractional oxygen concentration are necessary to obtain an adequate arterial saturation. Diuretics and fluid restriction may also be used to decrease preload. Inotropic agents such as digoxin are used to increase cardiac contractility, but their benefits are not clear if the indices of myocardial function are normal. Theoretically, when left ventricular dysfunction owing to chronic volume overload occurs, digoxin should be beneficial. Dobutamine and dopamine may be used in severe situations to improve cardiac output. If heart failure cannot be controlled with these measures, embolization of the cerebral arteriovenous shunts should be performed in the neonatal period.

Recently, the authors have identified a group of VGAM patients with severe heart failure and suprasystemic pulmonary hypertension who are resistant to nitric oxide and also have a lack of a clear-cut response to embolization. The exact treatment algorithm in these patients is yet to be determined. Recent studies suggest that management from the time of birth in the intensive care unit with mechanical ventilation and oxygen administration interferes with postnatal vascular lung maturation. This lack of normal pulmonary vascular remodeling may persist even after correction of the increased preload. Before starting treatment of the arteriovenous shunts, the patient's neurologic status needs to be assessed, and the cranial circumference, an electroencephalogram, and brain MR imaging need to be obtained.

The authors have developed a specific scoring system that takes into account neurologic, cardiac, respiratory, renal, and hepatic functions (Table 1). A total score of less than 8 is evidence of a poor systemic or neurologic outcome and may be an indication to withhold therapy. In the authors' series of patients, 25 of 140 newborns were not treated owing to severe brain damage, and 17 of 140 were not treated owing to multiorgan failure. Together, both groups of patients represent 17% of all infants and 30% of newborns managed at the authors' center. A score between 8 and 12 indicates a normal neurologic status but heart failure that is not responsive to medical treatment and the need for mechanical ventilation. Emergency embolization of the VGAM is mandatory in these patients. The goal of embolization is to reduce the arteriovenous shunting by one third, a proportion that results in improvement of systemic symptoms. Post embolization Doppler imaging reveals rapid improvement of cardiac and pulmonary functions, which allows for decreases in sedation and extubation of the infant. Mortality remains high, and neurologic scores are lower than in infants treated at 5 months of age. Neurologic assessment is difficult in neonates. Current

Table 1:   **Bicetre neonatal evaluation score**

Points	Cardiac function	Cerebral function	Respiratory function	Hepatic function	Renal function
5	Normal	Normal	Normal	—	—
4	Overload, no medical treatment	Subclinical isolated EEG abnormalities	Tachypnea, finishes bottle	—	—
3	Failure, stable with medical treatment	Nonconvulsive intermittent neurologic signs	Tachypnea, does not finish bottle	No hepatomegaly, normal function	Normal
2	Failure, not stable with medical treatment	Isolated convulsion	Assisted ventilation, normal saturation FiO_2 <25%	Hepatomegaly, normal function	Transient anuria
1	Ventilation necessary	Seizures	Assisted ventilation, normal saturation FiO_2 >25%	Moderate or transient hepatic insufficiency	Unstable diuresis with treatment
0	Resistant to medical treatment	Permanent neurologic signs	Assisted ventilation, desaturation	Abnormal coagulation, elevated enzymes	Anuria

Maximal score = 5 (cardiac) + 5 (cerebral) + 5 (respiratory) + 3 (hepatic) + 3 (renal) = 21.

methods to evaluate brain morphology and function do not permit identification of some injuries that may occur pre- or postnatally and do not become clinically evident until later. In the authors' series of over 140 neonates (including prenatally diagnosed cases), only 23 (among the 95 patients who were thought to have an acceptable neurologic prognosis) needed to be embolized during the neonatal age. One half of these patients died despite treatment.

A neonatal score between 13 and 21 allows one to delay the embolization of the malformation until the infant is 5 months of age. During the waiting period, the infant is followed up clinically, with special attention to cranial circumference because an increase may be the first indication of an unbalanced intracranial fluid state. Likewise, close neurologic and cardiac assessments are indicated to detect early symptoms arising in these organs. The authors suggest that MR imaging studies be obtained at birth and then at 3 months of age to evaluate myelination and morphologic cerebral status. Two thirds of patients referred to the authors did not need to be treated immediately but were able to wait until the optimal therapeutic window (5 months of age).

Unlike in prenatal patients and neonates, congestive heart failure is almost never the presenting symptom in infants, nor does it worsens at any age if already present. An increased cardiac index is often noted when the diagnosis of VGAM is made because of macrocrania. Most children need continuous treatment with diuretics until the time of embolization. After the first embolization, weaning from these medications is nearly always possible.

Neurologic manifestations

Intracranial venous hypertension resulting from the VGAM in combination with anatomic (the status of the cavernous sinuses and the degree of development of the base of the skull) and physiologic features (nonfunctioning pacchionian granulations) of the neonatal brain are the cause of neurologic deterioration [20,25,26]. Cerebral maturation requires a normal venous system capable of maintaining a fluid balance among the intracellular, extracellular, intraventricular, and intravascular spaces. Symptoms in fetuses or neonates are generally the result of intracranial venous congestion or hemodynamic alterations owing to heart failure during intrauterine life and reflect early brain damage. MR imaging (Fig. 12) may show focal white matter lesions or diffuse destruction of the brain (the melting brain), which is generally associated with severe cardiac insufficiency. These patients have low clinical scores, which is further evidence that aggressive treatment may not be indicated. In

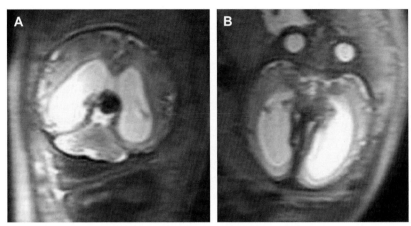

Fig. 12. (*A, B*) Prenatal MR imaging views in a fetus with a vein of Galen malformation showing parietal occipital brain areas of abnormal T2 hyperintensity and subependymal atrophy.

the authors' series, 25 of 140 patients showed zones of encephalomalacia, and 17 had low scores, both leading to a decision not to treat.

In infants, macrocrania may be the first objective clinical sign of an abnormal central nervous system. An increasing head circumference is commonly associated with enlarged ventricles and generous perivascular spaces in patients with VGAMs. This fluid accumulation has little or no effect on the brain as long as the sutures enlarge, resulting in a balance between the intracranial pressure and the resistance of the cranial vault. Macrocrania is the result of this adaptation and is possible as long as the skull sutures are patent. The cerebrofugal medullary veins form a gradient that will induce absorption of most of the intracerebral water. If the sutures close, if medullary vein resorption decreases as a result of increased pial venous pressure, or if for any other unknown reason the compliance of the venous system fails, hydrocephalus and intracranial hypertension occur (Fig. 13).

An unbalanced state of intracranial fluids and hydrocephalus are readily detected by consecutive measurements of head circumference and imaging studies. When hydrocephalus develops before the optimal date for embolization (5 months), embolization needs to be considered before placement of a CSF shunt or a ventriculostomy. CSF shunting does not address the underlying problem and results in transient and, often, incomplete resolution of hydrocephalus. CSF shunting creates a pattern of cerebropetal flow along the medullary veins that is opposite to the natural one (cerebrofugal). Following embolization, re-establishment of the cranial growth curve and a return to a normal state of intracranial fluid dynamics is observed (Fig. 14). In some instances, older children will eventually need a shunt despite adequate embolization.

Endoscopic ventriculostomy offers an acceptable alternative to ventricular shunt drainage after embolization in patients with a symptomatic hydrodynamic disorder in whom the basal arteries and veins are not significantly enlarged at the level of the expected ventriculostomy. Shunt-related complications such as intracerebral bleeds and subdural fluid/blood collections may be avoided by an understanding of their etiology and physiology and by carefully selecting patients in whom this type of treatment is truly necessary.

Developmental and psychomotor delays may also be related to cerebral venous disorders. Evidence of such problems is demonstrated by tests generally administered by pediatric neurologists. The authors' team uses the Denver or Brunet-Lezine tests [27] for these purposes. The difference between chronologic and apparent ages on testing is the basis for the diagnosis of neurocognitive delay. A 20% developmental delay is significant and may never be completely reversible. Below this 20% level, most embolized children will reverse to a normal neurocognitive state. The authors have developed a clinical score (Bicetre Admission and Outcome Score) to evaluate the neurologic clinical status (Table 2).

Many neurologic symptoms or cerebral hemorrhages in VGAM patients are secondary to ventricular shunting or treatment before or after the ideal therapeutic time window. The sequelae of these complications manifest as cerebral calcifications or subcortical and subependymal atrophy. The authors' treatment algorithm takes into account these complications. The goal is to anticipate and avoid them while minimizing the risk inherent to treatment. Morbidity and mortality are less in infants weighing greater than 5 kg than in newborns. As mentioned previously, embolization during the

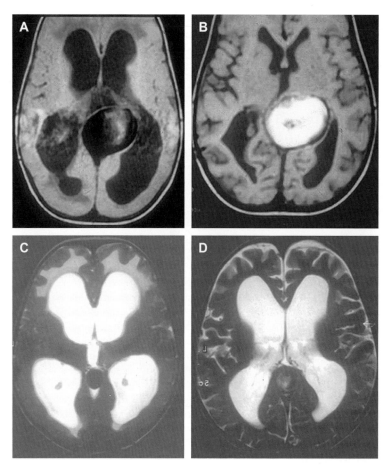

Fig. 13. (*A*) Axial T1-weighted image before embolization of a vein of Galen malformation with ventriculomegaly. (*B*) After embolization, an axial T1-weighted image shows occlusion of the malformation (high signal due to thrombus) and resolution of the hydrocephalus without use of ventricular shunting. (*C*) T2-weighted image before embolization shows ventriculomegaly with transependymal fluid resorption. After embolization (*D*), the interstitial edema is reduced and the ventricles have decreased in size.

first month of life is indicated only when the cardiac status of the patient is tenuous. Careful clinical and imaging follow-up allows these children to grow and permits one to delay the embolization until the optimal time window.

Therapeutic strategies

The goals of treatment are to improve existing clinical symptoms and avoid the development of new ones; therefore, these goals are different according

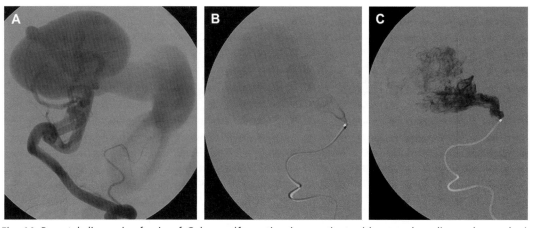

Fig. 14. Prenatal diagnosis of vein of Galen malformation in a patient with normal cardiac and neurologic growth. (*A*) Lateral view from the arterial phase of a vertebral artery injection demonstrating a mural type of malformation with single high-flow communication supplied by a posterior choroidal artery. (*B*) Selective catheterization of the fistula in frontal view. (*C*) Injection of undiluted histoacryl mixed with tantalum powder is shown in this view.

Table 2:	Bicetre admission and outcome score
Score	**Condition**
5	Normal (N)
4	Minimal non-neurologic symptoms, not treated (MS) and/or asymptomatic enlargement of the cardiac silhouette
3	Transient neurologic symptoms, not treated (TNS) and/or asymptomatic cardiac overload under treatment
2	Permanent minor neurologic symptoms, mental retardation of up to 20%; nonpermanent neurologic symptoms under treatment (MNS); normal school with support and/or cardiac failure stabilized with treatment
1	Severe neurologic symptoms, mental retardation of more than 20% (SNS); specialized school and/or cardiac failure unstable despite treatment
0	Death (D)

Does not apply to neonates.

to the age of the patient. In newborns, improvement of heart failure is the main goal, whereas in older children the goal is to prevent neurologic symptoms. For the authors, complete obliteration of the VGAM is not the main treatment goal, particularly when the therapy may result in morbidity and mortality. Treatment is based on a balance between technical difficulties (the weight of the child at the time of treatment) and the development of neurologic symptoms. In newborns, treatment is indicated when heart failure is refractory to medical treatment and when it prevents normal feeding and weight gain. Embolization is then performed after the first week of life to allow the infant's circulatory system to adapt to its new postnatal requirements. At this time, the goal of embolization is to reduce heart failure to a level at which the cardiopulmonary systems are performing as normal as possible.

In the authors' experience, reduction of about 30% of shunt volume rapidly improves cardiac status and permits the infant to be weaned off the ventilator. Afterward, embolization may be completed at 5 months of age. If embolization is still incomplete at that time, other sessions may be scheduled depending on the clinical evolution. On average, 2.5 treatment sessions per child are needed.

Angiographic criteria have permitted the authors to establish a treatment algorithm including the scheduling of future embolizations. Favorable venous findings that allow us to stage a procedure include the presence of an epsilon vein, use of the cavernous sinuses for cerebral drainage, mature venous sinuses at the base of the skull, patency of the jugular bulbs, and absence of reflux into the superior sagittal and superior petrosal sinuses.

Outside of heart failure in neonates, there are other situations in which emergent embolization may be required. The development of hydrocephalus implies that the CSF absorption mechanism has decompensated and is generally an indication for urgent embolization (Fig. 15). Ventricular shunting should be done after the embolization when the hydrocephalus is severe or irreversible. In infants, a rapid increase in head circumference even in the absence of other clinical signs and symptoms may be an indication for urgent embolization.

The venous route is associated with higher morbidity [28–31], and it should be used only when an arterial route is not available, when the clinical evolution deteriorates, or when the venous system shows a configuration that contains elements that place the patient at risk. Opacification of choroidal veins should be looked for in the venous phase of the vertebral artery angiogram. Visualization of the choroidal venous system is a contraindication to complete exclusion of the dilated venous pouch. In such patients, partial coil embolization may be indicated. In the authors' series of patients, the venous route was used in 5% of cases.

In the authors' opinion, radiotherapy is never indicated for the treatment of VGAMs. In our series, four children had radiotherapy [32], three before they were referred to us. In all three patients, a linear accelerator was used with no effect on the lesion; these three patients were subsequently cured by embolization. One other patient completed treatment with a combination of multi-focused radiotherapy following embolization of 80% of the lesion. The need for a long waiting period before the effects of radiotherapy take place leaves these infants at risk for complications related to acute or subacute venous ischemia.

Surgery has a role in the treatment of VGAMs but is mostly confined to the placement of ventriculostomies or ventriculoperitoneal shunting. Using

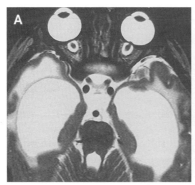
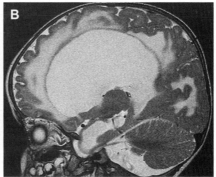

Fig. 15. (*A*) Axial T2-weighted image shows fluid surrounding the optic nerves and protrusion of the optic nerve heads into the vitri. (*B*) Parasagittal T2-weighted image shows hydrocephalus with transependymal fluid resorption in a child with a vein of Galen malformation and severe hydrodynamic disturbances.

Johnston's 1987 review [13,28] as a reference, the results of surgery in the management of VGAM were very poor, with a 38% to 91% mortality rate in all patients and a 33% to 77% mortality rate in the group of patients who received only surgery. Normal children represented only 4% to 32% of the entire patient cohort depending on the age group. These results are quite different from the results published for over 120 patients treated by transarterial embolization, which resulted in a 26% overall mortality rate. Seventy-eight percent of the children demonstrated a normal neurologic status on follow-up.

Spontaneous thrombosis of a VGAM is rare. In the authors' experience, 2.5% of patients show spontaneous thrombosis, but only one half of them are neurologically normal, which is less than what can be accomplished with proper treatment. Spontaneous thrombosis should not be considered a favorable outcome, and expecting it to occur does not represent an acceptable therapeutic strategy.

Technical issues

The authors approach VGAMs via a transarterial femoral route and do not use either brachial or cervical punctures. During the neonatal period, a weak pulse (due to cardiac failure) may make a femoral puncture difficult. On rare occasions, the use of Doppler sonography is needed to localize the femoral artery if the pulse is so weak that it is not palpable. In high-flow lesions in newborns, the authors use the Baltacci P1, 8 (Balt Extrusion, Montmorency, France), which is a catheter especially designed for high blood flow lesions in infants. This microcatheter is used directly through a 4-F sheath without a guiding catheter. In nearly all neonatal and infant patients, there is no need to use a coaxial system. This technique also minimizes fluid overload in children who already have heart failure. The amount of contrast used is 6 mL/kg. Our

angiographic protocol includes frontal and lateral views of the dominant vertebral artery injection. Patency of the jugular bulbs and the degree of venous sinus development at the base of the skull are studied, particularly on frontal views. Both internal carotid arteries are studied with lateral projections, with special attention to the presence or absence of the epsilon vein and drainage of the sylvian veins into the cavernous sinuses. Embolization is performed with nondiluted histoacryl mixed with tantalum powder for high-flow fistulas (Fig. 16) or mixed with Lipiodol when used to embolize the choroidal arterial pedicles. We do not use particles, balloons, or coils via the arterial route. The high rate of morbidity and mortality limit use of the transvenous approach. In the few (5%) transvenous cases treated, the authors have used mostly coils and occasionally glue.

After near-complete or complete occlusion of the lesion, the patient is kept sedated and intubated in the intensive care unit for 24 hours. The day after the embolization, the patient is woken up and weaned gradually. An average of 2.4 sessions per child are needed to obtain the expected therapeutic goal. Endovascular treatment sessions are scheduled every 3 to 6 months depending on the clinical status of the child and their response to the prior embolization.

Clinical results

Of 317 patients with VGAM who were aged less than 16 years and evaluated by the authors, 233 (73.5%) received embolization. In 67 patients (21.1%), the decision was made not to treat, and 17 (5.4%) patients were lost to follow-up. Of the patients who were not treated, 45 were newborns with areas of encephalomalacia or clinical scores less than 8 points. Of 16 untreated infants, nine showed areas of encephalomalacia, six had spontaneous occlusion of the lesion, and one remained unoperated owing to technical difficulties. In three fetuses,

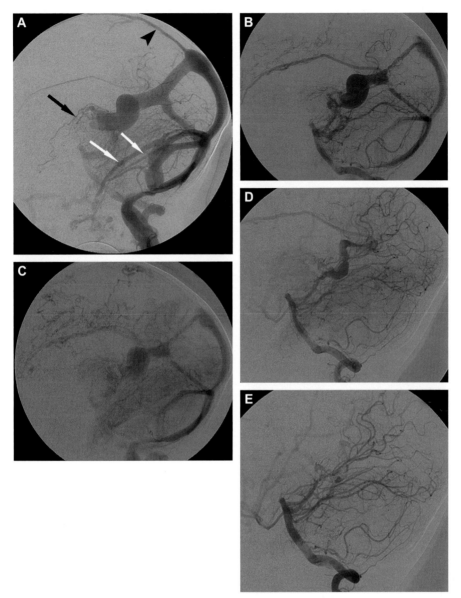

Fig. 16. Findings in a 12-month-old child previously undiagnosed who presented with macrocrania and facial venous dilatation from the age of 8 months and a mild degree of psychomotor retardation. (*A*) Lateral view of a vertebral artery injection shows a vein of Galen malformation with reflux into the choroidal veins (*black arrow*), superior sagittal sinus (*arrowhead*), and superior petrosal sinuses (*white arrows*). (*B–C*) Lateral view from a vertebral artery injection 1 year after partial embolization shows resolution of reflux into the choroidal veins, superior sagittal sinus, and superior petrosal sinuses but development of a spontaneous thrombosis of the right and falcine sinuses resulting in an unusual type of reflux into the inferior sagittal sinus and cortical veins that necessitated emergent occlusion of the shunt that was performed in two subsequent sessions (*D*) after the first session, and (*E*) after the last session.

termination of the pregnancy was chosen. Of infants older than 2 years of age, three had a clinical score of less than 1, two showed spontaneous occlusion, and the other had been previously treated with surgery. Embolization was employed in 88 newborns, 103 infants, and 42 older children (Table 3).

In the newborn group, 36.4% of those who were treated and are alive have had a normal neurologic development, 54.5% have a moderate degree of psychomotor maldevelopment, and 9.1% have a severe degree. In the newborn group, the overall mortality rate was 52%. Many of these patients presented at the beginning of the authors' experience, and, today, we would score them as 8 or less; therefore, they would fall into the nontreatment group. Current management strategies allow

Table 3: **VGAM therapeutic decision and proposed treatment**

	Embolization[a]	Abstention	Lost to follow-up	Total
Neonates	88 (5)	45	7	140
Infants	103 (8)	16	6	125
Children	42 (4)	6	4	52
Total	233 (17), 73.5%	67, 21.1%	17, 5.4%	317

[a] Numbers in parentheses denote embolization elsewhere.

for the identification of severe neonatal congestive heart failure, particularly that associated with treatment-resistant suprasystemic pulmonary arterial hypertension. These patients will have a poor prognosis despite emergent VGAM embolization.

In the infant patient group, 78.9% are now neurologically normal, 11.3% show a moderate degree of psychomotor development, and 9.8% show a severe one. The morbidity rate despite or due to embolization was 7.2%. In children over 2 years of age, 67.5% are neurologically normal, 20% show a moderate degree of psychomotor development, and 12.5% show a severe one. Procedure-related mortality was zero in the older age group. In patients in this group, neurologic symptoms were present before embolization and were probably related to the fact that treatment was given beyond the window of opportunity (Table 4).

Of the 193 embolized children who are alive, three sustained transient neurologic complications and four sustained permanent ones. Eleven children (5.7%) had post embolization hemorrhagic complications. Two children treated by the transvenous route after failure to achieve further embolization via the transarterial approach sustained an intracerebral hemorrhage within a few hours after the procedure. In both patients, occlusion of the venous outlet was complete while the flow into the VGAM was insufficiently reduced. From what has been reported in the literature [29–32] and based on the authors' limited experience with the transtorcular approach, hemorrhage occurs in more than 10% of cases after coil deposition.

After applying selection criteria, treatment was withheld in 18% of the children in the authors' series. The overall mortality rate in the group of embolized children was 10.6% (23 of 216 patients). The overall mortality rate for untreated and treated children was 23.7%.

Non-neurologic complications related to the embolization procedure or to the technical difficulty of injecting pure liquid adhesive occurred in 6.7% of patients. On three occasions, a drop of glue caused an asymptomatic partial occlusion of the internal iliac artery during removal of the catheter. All three patients showed progressive reconstitution of the vessel lumen on follow-up studies. In one additional patient, the catheter was glued in place intracranially, resulting in homonymous hemianopsia from which he recovered at 3 years' follow-up. In such a situation, the catheter should be cut as short as possible at the femoral entrance and pushed forward into the aorta where it rapidly becomes extraluminal and is incorporated into the vessel wall. This practice does not lead to any thrombotic or embolic manifestations in the authors' experience, nor does it require preventive anticoagulation. In a 4.6-kg baby girl, an aortotomy was deemed necessary to remove the catheter and a drop of glue in its tip that was considered too large to be removed through the sheath. The patient's postoperative course was uneventful. None of our patients have shown asymmetry in the growth of their lower extremities or other complications thought to be due to repeated femoral punctures.

Table 4: **Therapeutic results in the embolized VGAM group, 1981–2002**

Results	Neonates	Infants	Children	Total
Neurologically normal, BOS 3,4,5	36.4% (4/11)	78.9% (112/142)	67.5% (27/40)	74.0% (143/193)
Moderately retarded, BOS 2	54.5% (6/11)	11.3% (16/142)	20.0% (8/40)	15.6% (30/193)
Severely retarded, BOS 1	9.1% (1/11)	9.8% (14/142)	12.5% (5/40)	10.4% (20/193)
Death despite or due to embolization	52.0% (12/23)	7.2% (11/153)	0% (0/40)	10.6% (23/216)

Nearly 50% of neonates referred for management died. Many of these patients represent earlier cases that, today, would be scored below 8 and thus fall into the nontreatment group.
Abbreviation: BOS, Bicetre Outcome Score.

Morphologic results

In the group of 193 embolized children who are alive, 82 showed complete shunt obliteration, 55% showed a reduction of the shunt volume between 90% and 100%, 38.5% showed a reduction of 50% to 90%, and 6.2% showed a reduction of less than 50%. This last subgroup of patients is currently still undergoing treatment. Subtotal occlusions without choroidal or subependymal venous reflux (with minimal hemorrhagic, neurologic, or neurocognitive risks) are not completely treated if we believe that their procedure-related morbidity will be high. In 97% of the patients in whom treatment of the lesion was considered complete, total exclusion of the shunt was obtained and confirmed. In only 3% was the exclusion incomplete, and these infants are currently being observed with MR imaging and angiography.

Follow-up

Follow-up was obtained in children with complete shunt occlusion after embolization at 6 months. In the authors' series, the shunt remained closed in all patients. Once this anatomic cure is documented, the children are followed up clinically by a pediatric neurologist, and MR imaging is performed every 2 years. In the pediatric population, therapeutic success can only be truly evaluated when brain maturation is complete and functionally evaluated over time. Patients with subtotal or partial occlusions are followed up clinically and by MR imaging at closer intervals.

The status of the cardiac function is also observed closely. After embolization, the need for treatment of heart failure in newborns is diminished and is rare in infants. Discontinuation of this treatment is the prerogative of the cardiologist because it requires clinical and echocardiographic evaluations.

Summary

Based on their large group of patients with VGAM, the authors have concluded the following:

Although different types of malformations share a dilated vein of Galen, only one of them is a true VGAM.

The patterns of venous drainage are important in selecting the time of treatment. The optimal window of opportunity for treatment is between 4 and 5 years of age, because this allows the child to grow and mature.

Heart failure and hydrocephalus respond favorably to embolization. CSF ventricular shunting, if needed, should be performed after the embolization.

The transvenous approach carries significantly elevated morbidity and mortality and is rarely indicated.

Anatomic cure of the VGAM is not the main goal of treatment; the ultimate goal is control of the malformation to allow the brain to mature and develop normally and the child to grow healthy.

References

[1] Dandy WE. Cerebrospinal fluid: absorption. Chicago: American Medical Association; 1929. p. 2012.

[2] Boldrey E, Miller ER. Arteriovenous fistula (aneurysm) of the great cerebral vein (of Galen) and the circle of Willis. Arch Neurol Psychiatry 1949;62:147–70.

[3] Litvak J. Aneurysms of the great vein of Galen and midline cerebral arteriovenous anomalies. J Neurosurg 1960;17:945–54.

[4] Raimondi A. Vascular diseases. In: Raimondi A, editor. Pediatric neuroradiology. Philadelphia: Saunders; 1972. p. 629–42.

[5] Clarisse J. Aneurysms of the great vein of Galen: radiological-anatomical study of 22 cases. J Neuroradiol 1978;5(1):91–102.

[6] Diebler C. Aneurysms of the vein of Galen in infants aged 2 to 15 months: diagnosis and natural evolution. Neuroradiology 1981;21(4):185–97.

[7] Raybaud CA, Strother CM, Hald JK. Aneurysms of the vein of Galen: embryonic considerations and anatomical features relating to the pathogenesis of the malformation. Neuroradiology 1989;31:109–28.

[8] Pollock A. Cerebral arteriovenous fistula producing cardiac failure in the newborn infant. J Pediatr 1958;53:731–6.

[9] Claireaux AE. Arteriovenous aneurysm of the great vein of Galen with heart failure in the neonatal period. Arch Dis Child 1960;35:605–12.

[10] Glatt BS. Cerebral arteriovenous fistula associated with congestive heart failure in the newborn: report of two cases. Pediatrics 1960;26:596–603.

[11] Gold AP. Vein of Galen aneurysmal malformation. Acta Neurol Scand 1964;11(40):5–31.

[12] Amacher AL. The syndromes and surgical treatment of aneurysms of the great vein of Galen. J Neurosurg 1973;39(1):89–98.

[13] Johnston IH, Whittle IR, Besser M, et al. Vein of Galen aneurysmal malformation: diagnosis and management. Neurosurgery 1987;20:747–58.

[14] Lasjaunias P. Vascular diseases in neonates, infants and children: interventional neuroradiology management. Berlin: Springer; 1997.

[15] Lasjaunias P. Vascular diseases in neonates, infants and children: interventional neuroradiology management. 2nd edition. Berlin: Springer; 2007. in press.

[16] Fournier D, Rodesch G, Ter Brugge K, et al. Acquired mural (dural) arteriovenous shunt of the vein of Galen: report of 4 cases. Neuroradiology 1991;33:185–92.

[17] Lasjaunias P, Ter Brugge K, Lopez Ibor, et al. The role of dural anomalies in vein of Galen aneurysms: report of six cases and review of the literature. AJNR Am J Neuroradiol 1987;8:185–92.

[18] Okudera T, Huang YP, Ohta T, et al. Development of posterior fossa and radiologic study. AJNR Am J Neuroradiol 1994;15(10):1871–3.

[19] Girard N, Lasjaunias P, Taylor W, et al. Reversible tonsillar prolapse in vein of Galen aneurysmal malformations: report of eight cases and pathophysiological hypothesis. Childs Nerv Syst 1994;10:141–7.

[20] Zerah M, Garcia-Monaco R, Rodesch G, et al. Hydrodynamics in vein of Galen aneurysmal malformations. Childs Nerv Syst 1992;8:111–7 [discussion: 117].

[21] Chevret L, Durand P, Alvarez H, et al. Severe cardiac failure in newborns with VGAM: prognosis significance of hemodynamic parameters in neonates presenting with severe heart failure owing to vein of Galen arteriovenous malformation. Intensive Care Med 2002;28:1126–30.

[22] Rodesch G, Hui F, Alvarez H, et al. Prognosis of antenatally diagnosed vein of Galen aneurysmal malformations. Childs Nerv Syst 1994;10:79–83.

[23] Garcia-Monaco R, De Victor D, Mann C, et al. Congestive cardiac manifestations from cerebrocranial arteriovenous shunts: endovascular management in 30 children. Childs Nerv Syst 1991;7:48–52.

[24] Frawley GP, Dargaville PA, Pitchell PJ, et al. Clinical course and medical management of neonates with severe cardiac failure related to vein of Galen aneurysmal malformation. Arch Dis Child Fetal Neonatal Ed 2002;87(2): F144–9.

[25] Andeweg J. Intracranial venous pressures, hydrocephalus and effects of cerebrospinal fluid shunts. Childs Nerv Syst 1989;5:318–23.

[26] Taylor WJ, Hayward RD, Lasjaunias P, et al. Enigma of raised intracranial pressure in patients with complex craniosynostosis: the role of abnormal intracranial venous drainage. J Neurosurg 2001;94:377–85.

[27] Frankenburg WK, Dodds J, Archer P, et al. The Denver II: a major revision and restandardization of the Denver Developmental Screening Test. Pediatrics 1992;89:91–7.

[28] Mickle JP, Quisling RG. The transtorcular embolization of vein of Galen aneurysms. J Neurosurg 1986;64:731–5.

[29] Dowd CF, Halbach VV, Barnwell SL, et al. Transfemoral venous embolization of vein of Galen aneurysmal malformations. AJNR Am J Neuroradiol 1990;11:643–8.

[30] Charafeddine L, Numaguchi Y, Sinkin RA. Disseminated coagulopathy associated with transtorcular embolization of vein of Galen aneurysm in a neonate. J Perinatol 1999;19: 61–3.

[31] Lylyk P, Vinuela F, Dion JE, et al. Therapeutic alternatives for vein of Galen vascular malformations. J Neurosurg 1993;78:438–45.

[32] Watban JA, Rodesch G, Alvarez H. Transarterial embolization of vein of Galen aneurysmal malformation after unsuccessful stereotactic radiosurgery: report of three cases. Childs Nerv Syst 1995;11(7):406–8.

ELSEVIER
SAUNDERS

NEUROIMAGING
CLINICS
OF NORTH AMERICA

Neuroimag Clin N Am 17 (2007) 207–221

Diagnosis and Endovascular Treatment of Pediatric Spinal Arteriovenous Shunts

S. Cullen, MD[a], T. Krings, MD, PhD[b],*, A. Ozanne, MD[c],
H. Alvarez, MD[c], G. Rodesch, MD, PhD[c], Pierre Lasjaunias, MD, PhD[b,c]

Spinal arteriovenous shunts (SAVSs) are distinctly uncommon lesions in all age groups, but presentation in infants and children is rarer still. When SAVSs are diagnosed in pediatric patients, they are frequently associated with significant morbidity and their treatment is often challenging. The SAVSs seen in infants and children are not generally unusual or unique lesions from a morphologic standpoint, however. Early presentation of a SAVS in an infant or child may thus represent a particularly severe manifestation of disease processes that more commonly present in older patients. In other words, the SAVSs seen in the pediatric population may represent a more complete phenotypic expression of defects affecting the spinal circulation that manifest more frequently in a delayed and isolated manner. Seen in this light, the topic of this review—an analysis of the features that lead to early presentation of a SAVS in an infant or child less than 16 years of age—may shed light not only on SAVSs in the pediatric population but on all SAVSs, including those presenting in adults.

[a] Department of Radiology and Neurosurgery, Brigham and Women's Hospital, Francis Street, Boston, MA 02115, USA
[b] Department of Neuroradiology, University Hospital of the Technical, University Hospital Aachen, Pauwelsstrasse 30, 52057 Aachen, Germany
[c] Service de Neuroradiologie Therapeutique, CHU Bicêtre, 78 Rue du General Leclerc, 94275 Le Kremlin Bicêtre, CEDEX, France
* Corresponding author.
E-mail address: tkrings@izkf.rwth-aachen.de (T. Krings).

1052-5149/07/$ – see front matter © 2007 Elsevier Inc. All rights reserved.
neuroimaging.theclinics.com

doi:10.1016/j.nic.2007.02.004

Incidence of pediatric spinal arteriovenous shunts

The true incidence of SAVSs is not known. It has been estimated that SAVSs comprise 10% of all central nervous system (CNS) arteriovenous shunts (AVSs) in patients of all ages [1,2]. The incidence of brain arteriovenous malformations (BAVMs) in North America is 1.34 per 100,000 persons, and SAVSs are identified annually in approximately 1 in 1 million patients [3]. Diagnosis of a SAVS in a child is even less frequent. In the senior author's series of SAVSs seen at the Bicêtre Hospital, an international referral center for pediatric neurovascular disease in Paris, France, children accounted for 5% of all patients with CNS AVSs [4]. Pediatric SAVSs comprised 20% of SAVSs in all ages seen by this same group [5]. This number varies significantly from institution to institution relative to referral patterns and, of course, does not necessarily reflect incidence in the population as a whole. Whatever the true incidence of these lesions, it is likely that SAVSs are generally underdiagnosed because of their variable presentation and the complexity of diagnosis.

Classification of pediatric spinal arteriovenous shunts

The spinal cord and its circulatory system are significantly older phylogenetically than the cerebral circulation. The basic plan of spinal circulation—a fused ventral longitudinal channel supplemented by a perimedullary pial network supplied by segmental aortic branches—has remained relatively stable and unchanged throughout the ontogeny of vertebrates and across species. Profound genetic, molecular, or signaling errors that disrupt the normal developmental pathways, vasculogenesis, and vessel assembly in the spine during embryogenesis are likely most often lethal (here, the extreme eloquence of spinal cord tissue relative to volume likely also plays a role), and thus do not achieve high penetrance in the population. This may be one reason for the relative rarity of anatomic variation in the spinal (as compared with the cerebral) vasculature and possibly provides one explanation why SAVSs occur infrequently there. Certainly, the incidence of aneurysms is dramatically lower in the spine compared with the cerebral circulation [6]. Whatever the reasons for their rarity, it is likely SAVSs are the result of a range of underlying biologic defects that result in a susceptibility to form a pathologic condition, such as an AVS, but that require one or two triggering events after embryogenesis to achieve complete phenotypic expression, as has been proposed for other CNS vascular lesions [7,8]. In fact, there is evidence that a biologic defect

is responsible for a large number of SAVSs, particularly those that present in the pediatric population. A recent series of SAVSs presenting in children younger than 2 years of age, for example, found that nearly two thirds of patients (62%) had evidence of a heritable genetic defect (hereditary hemorrhagic telangiectasia [HHT]) or a somatic nonheritable mutation (spinal arteriovenous metameric syndrome [SAMS]) (Fig. 1) [9].

Several classifications have been used since SAVSs were first recognized as a clinical entity in the late 19th century [10–15]. The classifications have been used inconsistently, and the terminology, which is primarily descriptive, is often confusing. The situation is similar to the inconsistent and imprecise descriptive nomenclature used previously to describe vascular birthmarks and vascular anomalies. In 1982, Mulliken and Glowacki [16] focused on the endothelial cell characteristics of malformations and hemangiomas, clarified terminology, and proposed a classification that was grounded in the vascular biology of these lesions. Likewise, any classification of SAVSs, if it is to lead to better comprehension of these lesions, help to predict their natural history, and guide their treatment, must attempt to incorporate the vascular biology of these diseases.

The classification of SAVSs used here is the result of a 25-year single-center experience by the senior author treating SAVSs at the Bicêtre Hospital and has been outlined in numerous articles and book chapters (Box 1) [4,5,8,17–20]. First, a biologic basis for the SAVS is established and characterized. This may be a heritable mutation, such as one of the genetic defects associated with HHT, or a presumed somatic mutation if multiple lesions are present in a pattern consistent with SAMS [21]. Klippel-Trenaunay and Parkes-Weber syndromes have also been associated with SAVSs, as have neurofibromatosis and Ehlers-Danlos syndrome type IV, among others [4,22,23]. In the latter, however, the arterial wall disease focuses the lesion on the mural rupture of an artery into a venous plexus rather than a postcapillary vessel disorder. If no known genetic defect is present and the SAVS is not related to trauma, it is assumed to be an isolated sporadic SAVS. It is likely some of these isolated and apparently sporadic SAVSs may represent incomplete phenotypic expression of an underlying but undiagnosed genetic or segmental syndrome. Next, the morphology of the shunt is analyzed. A SAVS may be a fistula, consisting of a direct connection between the artery and vein, or a nidus, in which an intervening network of vessels is present. Fistulae are further subdivided into microfistulae and macrofistulae. The term *angioarchitecture* describes not only the morphology of a SAVS at

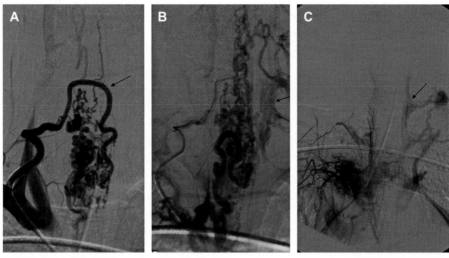

Fig. 1. SAMS involving the spinal myelomeres T2 and T3 and the nerve roots in a 17-year-old boy. (*A*) Spinal arteriovenous malformation (SAVM) is fed by a pial ventral network that arises from an enlarged anterior spinal artery (*arrow*), which, in turn, arises from the ascending cervical artery. (*B*) Venous drainage is directed caudally and cranially, and there is an outlet by way of the radicular veins into the epidural venous plexus (*arrow*). (*C*) In addition, a nerve root arteriovenous malformation (AVM) at the level of T3 on the right (*arrow*) can be appreciated after selective catheterization of the right T2/T3 artery. In SAMS (synonymous for Cobb syndrome), multiple AVMs may be present in a given metamere, which is defined as a functional developmental segment that includes skin, cartilage, muscle, vertebrae, peripheral nervous system, and central nervous system (CNS).

a given time but places the lesion in a temporal sequence, recognizing that most SAVSs induce changes over time; marked venous ectasias may develop, and additional arterial pedicles may be recruited. The type of shunt, nidus, or fistula, remains fixed; however, with time, some fistulae may resemble nidal type malformations because of the extensive pial reflux or intense intrinsic network congestion. Finally, the location of the SAVS is identified: intradural, epidural, or parachordal/paraspinal. Epidural lesions frequently include bone and may be malformations. So-called "spinal dural" AVSs are acquired and are excluded from this review because they relate to a different adult disease entity [19,20]. Intradural lesions may be superficial or deep in the cord. The type of shunt and its location have implications for the clinical presentation, treatment, and likelihood of complete cure with endovascular methods.

The pathophysiology of spinal cord arteriovenous shunts (SCAVSs) is poorly understood. Like BAVMs, they are not diagnosed antenatally, although they are congenital [7]. Most likely, a patient is born with a propensity to form an AVS, which then appears after a second or third event interferes with vessel repair or angiogenesis, although this process remains to be clarified. Presumably, etiologic factors important in the formation of BAVMs are also present in SAVSs. BAVMs are thought to represent populations of structurally unstable blood vessels with phenotypic evidence of upregulated angiogenesis [24]. Animal models suggest that errors in artery-vein identity, as dictated by the Notch signaling pathway, may also play a role [25]. Investigators have filled in some of the gaps in our knowledge of the pathophysiology of SAVSs with work done on the genetics, vascular biology, and endothelial cell biology of HHT in human beings and animal models.

Spinal cord arteriovenous lesions and hereditary hemorrhagic telangiectasia

HHT is an autosomal dominant disease with remarkably variable manifestations, including multifocal and multiorgan vascular dysplasias. Although classically defined by the triad of epistaxis, telangiectasias, and family history, patients with HHT can harbor AVSs in the pulmonary, hepatic, and CNS vasculature (Box 2, Tables 1 and 2) [26]. This disease is also likely underdiagnosed, but its prevalence is estimated to be between 1 in 5000 to 1 in 8000 persons, with clusters of higher prevalence in some Caribbean islands, Denmark, and the Jura region in Central Europe [27]. CNS involvement in this disease is common; up to 10% to 20% of individuals with HHT have BAVSs or SAVSs (Fig. 2) [28].

Mutations in three genes have been identified [29,30]. Most patients have mutations in the endoglin (ENG) or activin receptor-like kinase (ALK1) gene, both of which are members of the

Box 1:   Classifications of pediatric spinal cord arteriovenous shunts (intradural)

A. According to biologic abnormality

1. Heritable genetic defect

HHT type 1 (endoglin [ENG]) 9q33-34
HHT type 2 (activin receptor-like kinase [ALK1]) 12q11-14
HHT type 3 (Smad 4) 5q31-32

2. Nonheritable defect (somatic genetic) often segmental

SAMS
Klippel-Trenaunay syndrome with limb venolymphatic-associated lesions
Parkes-Weber syndrome

3. Sporadic isolated arteriovenous lesion (forme fruste of 1 and 2)
4. Acquired lesion (?)

B. According to morphology of AVS

Nidus (spinal cord arteriovenous malformation [SCAVM])
Fistula (spinal cord arteriovenous formation [SCAVF])

Macrofistula
Microfistula

Multifocal intradural lesions

C. According to location of SAVS

Intradural

Intramedullary
Extramedullary
Radicular
Filum

Epidural AVS (intraspinal)
Parachordal arteriovenous formation (AVF)

Branchial AVF
Vertebrovertebral arteriovenous formation (VVAVF)
Paraspinal arteriovenous formation (PSAVF)

Box 2:   Clinical diagnostic criteria for hereditary hemorrhagic telangiectasia

Nosebleeds, spontaneous and recurrent (rare in children)
Telangiectasias, multiple, at characteristic sites, including lips, oral cavity, fingers, and nose (rare in children)
Visceral lesions

Gastrointestinal telangiectasia (with or without bleeding)
Pulmonary arteriovenous malformation (AVM)
Hepatic AVM
Cerebral AVM
Spinal AVM

Family history: first-degree relative with HHT according to these criteria
Molecular DNA sequencing for endoglin (ENG) and activin receptor-like kinase (ALK1)
Many symptoms and signs of HHT may not be present until late in life

If two criteria are met, a diagnosis is possible; if three or more criteria are met, a diagnosis is definite.

Modified from Shovlin CL, Guttmacher AE, Buscarini E, et al. Diagnostic criteria for hereditary hemorrhagic telangiectasia (Rendu-Osler-Weber syndrome). Am J Med Genet 2000;91:66–7; with permission.

deficiencies in the cytoskeleton of the vessels. The first vessel segment affected seems to be the postcapillary venule, which supports the observation that, morphologically, these AVSs are a disease process centered in the venous circulation [7,31].

Table 1:   Clinical presentation of pediatric spinal arteriovenous shunts

Age	<2 years	<16years
M:F ratio	2:1	4:1
Hemorrhage	23%	70%
Weakness	62%	73%
Bruit	8%	NS
Sphincter	15%	27%
Asymptomatic	8%	17%
HHT	46%	17%
SAMS	15%	6%

Abbreviations: F, female; HHT, hereditary hemorrhagic telangiectasia; M, male; NS, not stated; SAMS, spinal arteriovenous metameric syndrome.
Data from Cullen S, Alvarez H, Rodesch G, et al. Spinal arteriovenous shunts presenting before 2 years of age: analysis of 13 cases. Childs Nerv Syst (in press); and Rodesch G, Hurth M, Ducot B, et al. Embolization of spinal cord arteriovenous shunts: morphological and clinical follow-up and results—review of 69 consecutive cases. Neurosurgery 2003;53:40–50.

transforming growth factor-β (TGFβ) pathway. TGFβ is a founding member of the largest family of secreted morphogens. TGFβ plays an important role in several processes during development and later, many of which include vessel assembly and angiogenesis [Mac Allister].

The HHT mutations seem to affect a pathway that induces proliferation, migration, and tube formation of endothelial cells, and disruption of this pathway has been shown to lead to deficient tube formation and poorly defined cord-like structures with weakened walls during angiogenesis [27]. The disorganized weak vessels may be a result of

Table 2: **Results of embolization of pediatric spinal arteriovenous shunts**

Age at presentation	<2 years	<16 years
Mean no. treatment sessions	2	1.5
Cured	78%	20%
>50% occluded	100%	100%
Complications (minor)	8%	10%
Complications (major)	0%	0%
Improved	75%	80%
Stable	25%	20%
Worse	0%	0%

Data from Cullen S, Alvarez H, Rodesch G, et al. Spinal arteriovenous shunts presenting before 2 years of age: analysis of 13 cases. Childs Nerv Syst (in press); and Rodesch G, Hurth M, Ducot B, et al. Embolization of spinal cord arteriovenous shunts: morphological and clinical follow-up and results—review of 69 consecutive cases. Neurosurgery 2003;53:40–50.

Specifically, excessive vascular endothelial growth factor (VEGF) expression in the setting of endoglin insufficiency may lead to the development of AVSs [32]. Interestingly, polymorphisms commonly seen in ALK1 (and possibly ENG) are associated with sporadic BAVMs [33].

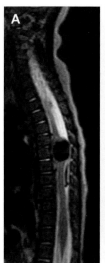
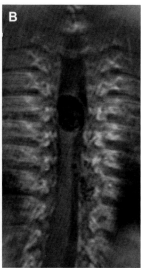

Fig. 2. MR imaging aspect of a single-hole arteriovenous fistula with a massively enlarged venous pouch that is located perimedullary, as seen in a sagittal T2-weighted image (*A*) and a coronal precontrast T1-weighted image (*B*). These lesions are high-flow arteriovenous macrofistulae that may become symptomatic because of venous congestion or mass effect. When encountered in a child, this aspect should always raise the suspicion of HHT (or Rendu-Weber-Osler disease).

In a recent review of 50 consecutive patients with HHT seen at the Bicêtre Hospital, a total of 75 CNS HHT-related vascular lesions were identified [34]. The mean age of the patients at presentation was 15 years. Seven patients had SAVSs, and all were fistulae (macrofistulae) [35]. In none of the patients were there multiple SCAVSs, although 1 patient had a SCAV fistula and two posterior fossa arteriovenous formations (AVFs). The age at presentation of patients with HHT and SAVSs was from 1 month of age to 6 years (mean = 2.2 years). Presenting symptoms included acute tetra- or paraplegia in 5 patients related to hematomyelia and progressive weakness in 2 patients, thought to be from subarachnoid hemorrhage in one and from venous congestion in the other. All lesions were macrofistulae located on the surface of the cord (perimedullary fistulae) and were supplied by the anterior spinal axis or radiculopial arteries. There were marked venous ectasias present, often with large venous pouches. Other authors have reported similar findings. In one early series of patients with spinal cord arteriovenous formations (SCAVFs), 2 of 10 patients had HHT [36]. Both of these patients were female and presented at 7 years of age, one with subarachnoid hemorrhage and lower extremity weakness and the other with acute paraplegia. Spinal angiography in both patients revealed macro-SCAVFs. Additional case reports discuss similar presentations: macro-SCAVFs in patients with HHT presenting as infants and young children [37,38]. In fact, although an identical lesion can be seen in children without HHT, the presence of a large single-hole macro-SCAVF in a young child is strongly suggestive of the diagnosis of HHT [9]. Some have proposed that this lesion be added to the criteria for the diagnosis of HHT [35].

Although the postcapillary venules seem to be type of blood vessel most severely affected by the biologic defect in HHT, the reduced level of endoglin is present in all endothelial cells throughout the body [27]. Although this leads to cutaneous manifestations, including telangiectasias, that appear in stereotypical locations (face, oral cavity, and hands), they are not distributed in a metameric pattern relative to the CNS abnormalities when present.

Spinal arteriovenous metameric syndromes and associated anomalies

A second group of patients with SAVSs shows evidence of a nonfamilial genetic defect that seems to affect vessels in a metameric pattern. A metamere is a functional developmental segment that includes skin, cartilage, muscle, peripheral nervous system elements, arteries, CNS, and visceral organs.

In the spine, the metamere is centered at the disc and includes half of the vertebral body above and half below. The presumed abnormality seen in SAMS may give rise to multiple lesions (again, all within the same metamere), but it is never heritable as a de novo somatic mutation. The first descriptions of this syndrome appear simultaneously with the early reports of SAVSs in the late 19th century, an era when the thorough physical examination was not yet supplanted by diagnostic imaging [39,40]. SAMS is likely much more common than the small number of case reports and case series would suggest [41–44]. The cutaneous malformation is often subtle and may be missed if not actively looked for. Fifteen percent of children presenting before 2 years of age with SAVSs in one recent series were found to have SAMS, and these patients were not symptomatic from their SAVSs at the time of diagnosis [9]. When all children seen at the Bicêtre Hospital are included, 10% had SAMS [4]. In another series, patients with SAMS comprised 21% of patients with SAVSs seen [41]. Vascular lesions may also be multifocal in a non-metameric distribution [42]. In another large series of SAVSs, 23% had associated vascular abnormalities [6].

By one estimate, as many as 28% of patients with SAVSs harbor associated vascular lesions, and among these, 10% are distributed in a metameric pattern [20]. Patients with multiple lesions not fitting a strict metameric distribution may represent a subset with incomplete phenotypic expression of the somatic defect(s), analogous to those with isolated solitary lesions. In one series of 19 patients with multifocal SAVSs and associated lesions, this group represented 16% of the patients with SAVSs seen at a single institution [42]. Within this group, there were nine cases of SAMS, four cases of Klippel-Trenaunay syndrome, and two cases of Parkes-Weber syndrome. Associated lesions included those vertebral lesions usually called hemangiomas, paraspinal arteriovenous shunts (PSAVSs), and cutaneous lesions (usually of the capillary-venous type). Interestingly, none of these patients had HHT.

Clinical presentation

Although heritable and nonheritable genetic abnormalities, such as HHT and SAMS, represent a significant number of pediatric patients with SAVSs, they nonetheless comprise the minority. Most patients do not meet the criteria for HHT, nor do they have the stigmata of a metameric vascular cutaneous lesion. Does the angioarchitecture of the SAVSs in these cases then explain the clinical presentation (**Figs. 3 and 4**)? Apart from the presence of a false aneurysm or pseudoaneurysm representing the likely source of bleeding (analogous to BAVMs), no clear correlation between angioarchitecture and symptoms was found in a large series of intradural SAVSs [5]. In this series, 30 patients (19%) were seen before the age of 15 years. There was a high male predominance (24 boys and 6 girls). In comparison, the male-to-female ratio almost

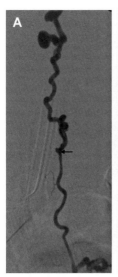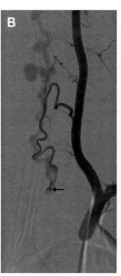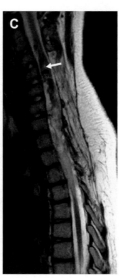

Fig. 3. At the age of 8 months, this 10-year-old boy was operated on at an outside institution because of the sudden onset of paraplegia attributable to spinal subarachnoidal and intramedullary hemorrhage. Control angiography after the intervention showed a residual fistula that was subsequently controlled on MR imaging. At the age of 9 years, the boy presented with acute pain and a new motor deficit of his upper limbs and was subsequently referred to our institution. Angiography revealed a perimedullary fistula at the level of T2 that was fed by a radiculopial branch of the left T4 intercostal artery (*A*) and the vertebral artery (*B*). The latter injection allowed us to pinpoint the exact transition of the artery into the vein (*arrow in A and B*) and, subsequently, to obliterate the fistula successfully by means of an endovascular approach with glue disposition at the most proximal venous and most distal arterial segments. (*C*) MR imaging revealed the sequelae of the old hemorrhage and thrombosis within the ecstatic venous channels (*arrow*).

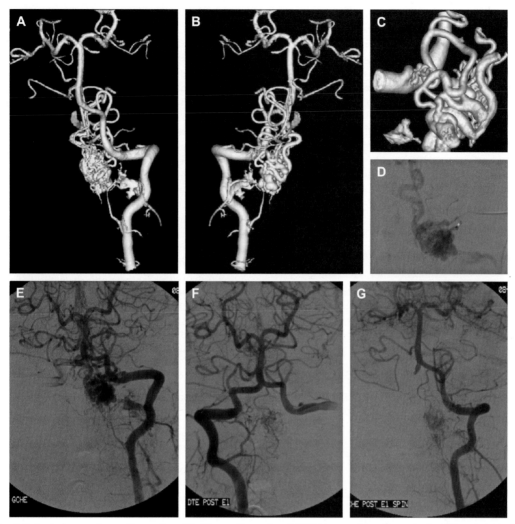

Fig. 4. Spinal glomerular malformation. The three-dimensional (3D) images show the anterior (*A*) and posterior (*B*) aspects of the malformation, and the enlarged posterior view (*C*) clearly demonstrates associated ectasias and intranidal aneurysms as potentially dangerous angioarchitectural areas that were subsequently embolized after superselective catheterization (*D*). Arteriovenous malformation (AVM) before (*E*) and after (*F, G*) embolization, with an important reduction in size and shunting volume and complete occlusion of the intranidal aneurysm.

attained parity in the adult population (65 male and 60 female patients). Most of the SAVSs were located in the cervical or thoracic spine. There were twice as many nidus type shunts as fistulae (20 spinal cord arteriovenous malformations [SCAVMs] and 10 SCAVFs). Importantly, 21 of the 30 patients presented with hemorrhage (11 with hematomyelia and 10 with subarachnoid hemorrhage). In general, children with hematomyelia developed a severe deficit at presentation; those patients with subarachnoid hemorrhage had milder symptoms. In the adult cohort, only 45% presented with hemorrhage. Those 9 pediatric patients who presented without hemorrhage had acute symptoms ascribed to venous congestion, with or without venous

thrombosis. Arterial steal was not thought to be the cause of symptoms. A statistical analysis did not show angioarchitectural features that could be used reliably to predict the risk of hemorrhage.

SAVSs in extremely young children form a special group akin to those in patients with vein of Galen malformations, dural sinus malformations, pial AVFs, and PHACES syndrome. The SAVS in these patients, however, is not a distinct anatomic entity; identical lesions can appear in older patients, including adults. In a series of 13 patients presenting with SAVSs before 2 years of age, 10 patients had intradural SAVSs and there were two epidural shunts and one paraspinal shunt [9]. The mean age at presentation was 7 months. A male predominance was again seen, with 9 boys and 4 girls. Of note, hemorrhagic presentation was significantly lower than in the age group younger than 15 years; it was seen in only 3 (23%) of the 13 patients. (In this study epidural and paraspinal shunts were included. If only intradural SAVSs are considered, hemorrhagic presentation was seen in 20% of patients). The relatively low rate of hemorrhage may be explained by the high proportion of high-flow macro-SCAVFs (77%), with symptoms ascribed to the severe pial reflux and venous hypertension of the spinal cord. As mentioned previously, there was an extremely high proportion of patients in this study with a syndromic association, with 8 (62%) of 13 patients found to have HHT or SAMS.

Epidural and paraspinal arteriovenous shunts

At first glance, epidural AVSs and PSAVSs may seem to represent a distinct set of disorders with little in common with the group of intradural SAVSs. Although a heterogeneous group of lesions, these SAVSs may be unified by their relation to the notochord [7]. The notochord is one of the first organs to develop in the vertebrate embryo, and it plays an important role as a mechanical structure necessary for locomotion as well as an axial signaling center crucial for the patterning of adjacent tissues, including nervous and vascular tissues [45]. Mutant animal model embryos lacking notochord fail to form a dorsal aorta and lack primary intersegmental vessels [46]. This group of SAVSs extends from the rostral extent of the notochord at the basisphenoid (cavernous sinus) caudally through the lumbar and sacral regions and includes branchial AVFs (maxillary artery-to-vein fistulae, ascending pharyngeal-to-jugular vein arteriovenous fistulae, and occipital-to-vertebral vein fistulae), the vertebrovertebral arteriovenous formations (VVAVFs) and other PSAVSs in the cervical, thoracic, and lumbar spine.

As with the intradural SAVSs, associated genetic or biologic defects may be identified in patients with this group of lesions. Neurofibromatosis I and collagen disorders are associated with VVAVFs with the nosologic restrictions mentioned previously, and an association with HHT, Klippel-Trenaunay-Weber syndrome, collagen disorders, and SAMS has already been noted [4,9,47–49]. The PSAVSs are then only detected fortuitously, or possibly by auscultation of a bruit. The proximity of large low-resistance venous outlets (internal jugular and azygos venous systems) can, if accessed by the adjacent AVF, create a situation in which cardiac overload may develop [7]. Centripetal drainage may also occur, however, with presentations similar to those discussed previously with intradural

SCAVSs, including subarachnoid hemorrhage [9,21].

In the head and neck region, the branchial AVSs include maxillary and pharyngeal AVFs. These children may present with a bruit (often imperceptible to them because it has been present from an early age) or a slowly enlarging pulsatile mass. Similarly VVAVFs have a bruit or pulsatile mass as the most frequent presenting symptom. Intradural or intracranial venous drainage is exceedingly rare in VVAVFs. Lower cervical VVAVFs may more commonly access the intradural venous system and produce pial congestion and cord symptoms [7,50]. Lower cervical and thoracic AVFs are not common in the pediatric population. Typically, these are high-flow lesions with centrifugal flow. Thoracolumbar PSAVSs are even less common in the pediatric population, and symptoms are usually minimal and indolent until venous drainage is rerouted centripetally. There should always be a high clinical suspicion for SAMS or HHT when confronted with these lesions. In one series of 10 cases of PSAVS (excluding VVAVF), one patient had neurofibromatosis and one had SAMS. Four patients presented before 15 years of age (2 boys and 2 girls) [51].

Diagnosis of spinal cord arteriovenous shunts

Noninvasive imaging

MR imaging is the preferred screening modality for evaluating SAVSs. Tissue contrast and anatomic resolution afforded by current standard MR imaging sequences are sufficient to make the diagnosis of a spinal arteriovenous malformation (SAVM) or paraspinal arteriovenous malformation (PSAVM) in most cases. Flow voids identified on T1- and T2-weighted sequences correspond to dilated draining veins and can be used to locate the site of the shunt in relation to the dura. With MR imaging, it can be difficult to differentiate extensive intradural venous distention associated with some epidural or paraspinal shunts reliably from an intradural shunt. Associated changes, including cord compression, cord edema, and hemorrhage (whether hematomyelia or subarachnoid), are usually readily apparent. Injection of gadolinium–diethylenetriamine penta-acetic acid (DTPA) may reveal cord enhancement, which has been attributed to venous stasis, ischemia, or infarction of the cord. It is seldom possible to distinguish spinal arteriovenous formations (SAVFs) from SAVMs using MR imaging. Small ventral shunts with draining veins in the ventral sulcus may remain occult on MR imaging [52,53]. The anatomic location of the nidus of the malformation and, often, the approximate location of the feeding arteries can be readily identified. In all cases, the entire spinal axis should be imaged. In the case of SAMS, associated lesions (eg, intramedullary, epidural, paraspinal, soft tissue) often can be seen. Spinal magnetic resonance angiography (MRA) may be performed to provide supplemental information but is not currently of adequate diagnostic accuracy that it may supplant spinal digital subtraction angiography (DSA). CT may be useful in evaluating bony erosion, which can help to localize large venous pouches that may be a target for transvenous embolization in certain paraspinal lesions, but this is rarely necessary; in general, CT does not contribute to the imaging assessment of spinal vascular lesions in this population. Although used frequently in the past, myelography does not currently have a role in the evaluation of patients suspected of having SAVSs (Fig. 5).

Spinal angiography

The primary imaging technique for the detailed evaluation of spinal vascular lesions after an MR imaging scan has been obtained and reviewed is selective spinal DSA. Spinal cord angiography is an invasive procedure that requires interventional expertise. The authors perform angiography regardless

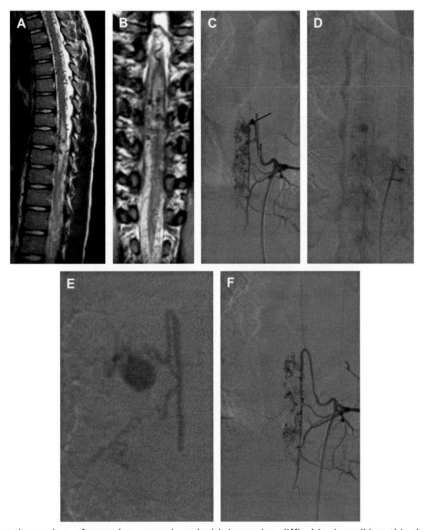

Fig. 5. During the workup of secondary enuresis and with increasing difficulties in walking, this glomerular intramedullary arteriovenous malformation (AVM) was identified that on MR imaging (*A, B*) and is consistent with intramedullary congestive edema and dilated perimedullary veins indicative of an arteriovenous shunt (*C*). On angiography, injection into the left T11 intercostal artery reveals an intranidal aneurysm (*arrow*) with persistence of contrast media in the late venous phase (*D*). (*E*) This intranidal aneurysm is subsequently superselectively catheterized and occluded with liquid embolic material. (*F*) Control after embolization with persistence of the anterior spinal artery and complete occlusion of the aneurysm.

of the age of the patient. The procedure is performed under general anesthesia, with femoral access by means of a 4- or 5-French sheath, depending on the patient's size. Selective injections are crucial for an accurate assessment of the angioarchitecture of a spinal vascular lesion. This includes identification of all feeding pedicles and analysis of draining veins. Vascularity of adjacent spinal cord should also be clearly demonstrated. Nonselective aortograms are never sufficient. Of note, the intradural spinal arteries in neonates and infants are proportionately larger and more tortuous than in the normal adult; this should not be interpreted as a pathologic finding. Demonstration of angiographically normal spinal vascular supply includes depiction of the venous drainage of the cord. Three-dimensional (3D) rotational spinal DSA can be useful in mapping the morphology of the SAVS. In particular, 3D spinal DSA is helpful in identifying intranidal pseudoaneurysms and in evaluating the feasibility of embolization (Fig. 6).

Natural history and choice of treatment of pediatric spinal cord arteriovenous shunts

Decisions regarding the relative risks and benefits of treatment of SAVSs as well as the timing of therapy depend on an understanding of the natural history of these lesions. Early case series reporting on the natural history of SCAVSs in patients of all ages supported the impression that the prognosis is extremely poor for patients with these lesions once they have developed symptoms. When SCAVFs are excluded, the natural history of SAVSs seems to be less severe than previously thought [20]. In the Bicêtre Hospital experience in the pediatric age group, fully 72% of patients with hemorrhagic presentation improved. Recurrent hemorrhage was seen in only 9% of patients (3.6% in adults). Only 20% had progressive worsening of symptoms. Similarly, in extremely young patients, there was no rehemorrhage [9]. Emergency treatment of these lesions does not therefore seem to be justified.

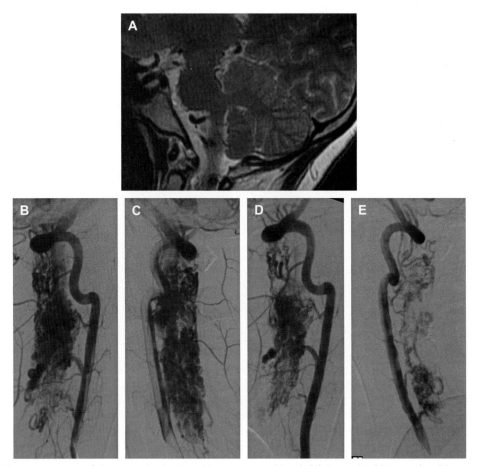

Fig. 6. Extensive SAVM of the cervical spinal cord in a 17-year-old girl. (*A*) On sagittal T2-weighted images, multiple dilated perimedullary and intramedullary flow voids can be seen. Angiography of both vertebral arteries (*B, C*) demonstrates the congestive aspect of the veins before embolization and the massive reduction of the venous congestion after superselective embolization (*D, E*).

Therapeutic strategy

The therapeutic strategy includes a clinical objective (eg, preventive, corrective, palliative) and related morphologic target and goal. The overall treatment may thereafter depend on the anatomy of the SAVS, which guides the technical choice. In general, SCAVFs have a high likelihood of complete cure, whereas SCAVMs, because of their more complex anatomy, are rarely obliterated without risk of deficit. Partial targeted embolization is a prudent compromise, improving on the natural history without putting the patient at risk for deterioration if the goal is complete cure. The degree of comfort with different treatment options likely differs among operators and from institution to institution, and the chosen therapy should most likely be performed, if at all possible, at a referral center with considerable experience in pediatric neurovascular surgery, interventional neuroradiology, and pediatric neurocritical care. In the authors' experience, most patients are best treated with endovascular techniques, or in certain cases, no treatment. When treatment is deemed necessary and the anatomy is unfavorable for an endovascular approach, a few patients are considered for open surgical treatment. At several centers, surgery is the primary treatment for SAVSs, with or without preoperative embolization. Results have been reported in several case series [2,15,54–57]. Although there are reports proposing a role for radiation therapy in the treatment of SCAVSs, the authors believe that radiation therapy for SCAVSs is not currently a viable alternative to other established methods.

Timing of therapy and technical remarks

Treatment of an SCAVS is almost never an emergency. In nearly all cases, a diagnostic procedure is recommended first to document the extent of the shunt and map the arterial supply and venous drainage. Patients with SCAVSs presenting with hemorrhage are nearly always permitted to recover from their hemorrhage before any intervention is performed. Surgery to decompress an acute hematomyelia can be deleterious. In general, the first embolization occurs 6 to 8 weeks after the initial event. Early or frequent rehemorrhage is not a typical feature of this disease, although differences may exist in extremely young patients. If the diagnostic angiogram reveals an arterial pseudoaneurysm associated with a ruptured SCAVM, partial targeted embolization may be considered, analogous to the approach outlined by the authors for ruptured BAVMs [58].

Historically, a variety of embolic agents have been used to treat SCAVSs, including liquid adhesives, polyvinyl alcohol particles, coils, and balloons. Particles are a temporary agent but may have a role in the preoperative embolization of SCAVSs, although the senior authors of this review have not used particles for the treatment of SCAVS in more than 25 years. With the exception of certain paraspinal shunts (eg, vertebrovertebral formations [VVFs]) in which balloons and or coils are used, N-butyl cyanoacrylate is the agent of choice. The role of ethylene-vinyl alcohol (EVOH) is currently not clear [59]. Important limitations to its applicability to the treatment of pediatric neurovascular disease of the spine include the toxicity of its solvent, dimethyl sulfoxide (DMSO), which is particularly of concern in low-weight patients, and the relative inflexibility of microcatheters currently approved for its delivery. In addition, EVOH may not be suitable for the high-flow type of shunts seen frequently in the spine in this age group. We consider it to be extremely dangerous in the spinal cord territories in relation to the size of the access arteries, the size of the target, the acute bends and tortuosity of the feeders, and the risk of wedged injections in the intrinsic network.

Over-the-wire catheters are seldom capable of negotiating the tortuous anatomy frequently encountered; thus, flow-directed microcatheters are used (1.2 and 1.5 French). Pathways to the site of the SCAVS include radiculopial (posterior spinal) and radiculomedullary (anterior spinal) arteries. The latter is used as a route to the sulcocommissural arteries, which may be safely embolized as long as caution is exercised not to interrupt the anterior spinal axis. Some authors endorse the use of spinal evoked potentials, with provocative testing with sodium amytal [20,60]. Hemodynamic manipulation, including such maneuvers as artificially lowering arterial blood pressure in extremely high-flow fistulae, can be helpful. As stated previously, SCAVMs, because of the complex anatomy of the nidus, are rarely completely obliterated with endovascular techniques. Exclusion of pseudoaneurysms and reduction of the flow and total size of the nidus, however, are thought to improve the natural history of the lesion at acceptable levels of risk. SCAVFs have less complex morphology and are frequently cured with endovascular techniques.

Treatment strategies for extradural SCAVSs are similar, with the goals being obliteration of the shunt and preservation of the parent vessels and the normal supply to the spinal axis. Liquid adhesive (N-butyl-cyanoacrylate) is, again, the primary embolic agent, although coils and balloons are used for some lesions. Specifically, detachable balloons (if available), alone or in combination with coils, provide efficient treatment for many parachordal lesions, wherein disconnection of the shunt and preservation of the parent vessel can usually be achieved. Recurrence can occur, and a transvenous approach has been recommended by some [50,61].

Epidural and paraspinal shunts are also amenable to endovascular techniques. Hui and colleagues [62] described treatment of two children with paraspinal arteriovenous formations (PSAVFs) with transarterial glue injections in both patients, supplemented by transvenous deposition of coils in one child. Goyal and colleagues [51] included four children younger than 15 years of age in their series of 10 PSAVFs. Three underwent treatment (transarterial) for thoracic and lumbar epidural fistulae, and a cure was achieved in all. One child with a thoracic epidural and bone arteriovenous malformation (AVM) was not treated. Typically, treatment of fistulae is straightforward. Epidural branches are usually accessible and safely embolized. Care must be taken to outline the normal supply to the spinal cord before proceeding with embolization, because significant contributions to the anterior spinal axis may be occult if adjacent to high-flow contributors to large shunts. As with embolization of fistulae at other sites, penetration past the actual site of shunting is mandatory. Incomplete transarterial embolization of large paraspinal shunts is equivalent to a proximal ligation. This does not provide an effective long-term benefit and may make subsequent treatment more difficult as other vessels are recruited to supply the fistula. Transvenous occlusion of a large recipient venous pouch with coils, liquid adhesive, or both can augment transarterial embolization and be an effective approach for some high-flow paraspinal fistulae [63]. Finally, glue may also be used to occlude extracranial parachordal shunts, including maxillary AVFs, but patency of the parent vessel as well as of cranial segmental vessels should be maintained if possible. Similarly, pharyngeal AVFs can be approached transarterially with this agent, but care must be taken when embolizing vessels in the vicinity of the jugular foramen, because cranial nerve damage may result (IX, X, XI, XII).

Apart from standard postoperative care and fluids, posttreatment management may include low-dose heparin if venous restrictive disease is noted and complete occlusion of the AVF is achieved. This is used to prevent possible extensive and rapid venous thrombosis. Embolization of normal arterial branches may result in significant pain, including radicular pain, muscular pain, and even trismus. This is managed symptomatically and is usually transient. Significant swelling of SCAVSs after embolization has not been observed.

Embolization of pediatric spinal cord arteriovenous shunts: results

The angiographic and clinical results of a large series of consecutive patients with intradural SCAVSs treated with embolization were reviewed by Rodesch and colleagues [18]. This series of 69 treated patients (of a series of 155 patients) included 20 children and 49 adults. In all patients, complete obliteration of SCAVSs was achieved in 16% and a reduction of more than 50% was seen in 86% of cases. No recanalization was seen at follow-up angiography (mean follow-up = 5.6 years). Outcomes were deemed good in 83% of patients, with 15% being asymptomatic, 43% improved, and 25% stable. No stabilization was achieved in 4%. Transient deficits were seen in 14% of patients, and permanent severe complications were seen in 4%. The response was particularly encouraging in the pediatric group, in which 16 (80%) of 20 patients undergoing embolization (versus 49% of adults) were clinically improved after treatment.

In the neonatal and infant group, the response to endovascular treatment was particularly good. In a series of 13 cases of SCAVS (intradural and extradural lesions) in children presenting before 2 years of age, eight patients underwent endovascular treatment alone and one had surgery and embolization [9]. Of those patients who were treated with embolization, complete obliteration of the lesion was achieved in seven and 90% reduction was achieved in two. In those treated patients with follow-up, seven of nine were improved and two of nine were stable. There was no permanent morbidity or mortality in this series.

In the series of PSAVSs of Goyal and colleagues [51], which included 4 pediatric patients of a total of 10 patients, 3 of the 4 pediatric patients underwent endovascular treatment using a combination of transarterial and transvenous methods. Complete obliteration of the fistulae was achieved in all cases.

Summary

The group of SAVSs that are diagnosed in neonates, infants, and children are not anatomically distinct from those that appear in older patients, but several important features are characteristic. There is a particularly high association with genetic abnormalities, including HHT and SAMS. These syndromes should be diligently sought for when confronted with a child with an SAVS. The predilection to affect male patients is more pronounced than in the adult cohort. A hemorrhagic presentation is much more frequent than in adults, except in extremely young children. The natural history seems to be better than previously thought, with spontaneous recovery after hemorrhage being the rule and rehemorrhage being rare. Although this group of lesions is the cause of significant morbidity, many SAVSs in children are amenable to endovascular therapy, often with excellent anatomic results and improvement or stabilization of symptoms.

References

[1] Stein BM. AVMs of the brain and spinal cord. In: Hoff JT, editor. Practice of surgery. New York: Harper & Row; 1979.

[2] Cogen P, Stein BM. Spinal cord arteriovenous malformations with significant intramedullary components. J Neurosurg 1983;59:471–8.

[3] Stapf C, Mast H, Sciacca RR, et al. The New York Islands AVM study: design, study progress and initial results. Stroke 2003;34:29–33.

[4] Rodesch G, Hurth M, Alvarez H, et al. Classification of spinal cord arteriovenous shunts: proposal for a reappraisal—the Bicetre experience with 155 consecutive patients treated between 1981 and 1999. Neurosurgery 2002;51:374–80.

[5] Rodesch G, Hurth M, Alvarez H, et al. Angio-architecture of spinal cord arteriovenous shunts at presentation. Clinical correlations in adults and children. Acta Neurochir (Wien) 2004;146:217–27.

[6] Hurth M, Houdart R, Djindjian R, et al. Arteriovenous malformations of the spinal cord: clinical, anatomical and therapeutic considerations—a series of 150 cases. Prog Neurol Surg 1978;9:238–66.

[7] Lasjaunias P. A revised concept of the congenital nature of cerebral arteriovenous malformations. Intervent Neuroradiol 1997;3:275–81.

[8] Lasjaunias P, ter Brugge K, Berenstein A. Spinal arteriovenous shunts. In: Surgical neuroangiography, vol. 3. Clinical and interventional aspects in children. 2nd edition. New York: Springer Verlag; 2006. p. 721–66.

[9] Cullen S, Alvarez H, Rodesch G, et al. Spinal arteriovenous shunts presenting before 2 years of age: analysis of 13 cases. Childs Nerv Syst (in press).

[10] Anson JA, Spetzler RF. Classification of spinal arteriovenous malformations and implications for treatment. BNI Q 1992;8:2.

[11] Bao YH, Ling F. Classification and therapeutic modalities of spinal vascular malformations in 80 patients. Neurosurgery 1997;40:75–81.

[12] Heros R, Debrun G, Ojemann RG, et al. Direct spinal arteriovenous fistula: a new type of spinal AVM. J Neurosurg 1986;64:134–9.

[13] Marsh WR. Vascular lesions of the spinal cord: history and classification. Neurosurg Clin N Am 1999;10:1–8.

[14] Merland JJ, Reizine D, Laurent A, et al. Embolization of spinal cord vascular lesions. In: Vinuela F, Halbach VV, Dion J, editors. Interventional neuroradiology: endovascular therapy of the central nervous system. New York: Raven Press; 1992. p. 153–65.

[15] Spetzler RF, Detwiler PW, Riina HA, et al. Modified classification of spinal cord vascular lesions. J Neurosurg 2002;96:145–56.

[16] Mulliken JB, Glowacki J. Hemangiomas and vascular malformations in infants and children: a classification based on endothelial characteristics. Plast Reconstr Surg 1982;69:412–22.

[17] Rodesch G, Hurth M, Alvarez H, et al. Spinal cord intradural arteriovenous fistulae: anatomic, clinical, and therapeutic considerations in a series of 32 consecutive patients seen between 1981 and 2000 with emphasis on endovascular therapy. Neurosurgery 2005;57:973–83.

[18] Rodesch G, Hurth M, Ducot B, et al. Embolization of spinal cord arteriovenous shunts: morphological and clinical follow-up and results—review of 69 consecutive cases. Neurosurgery 2003;53:40–50.

[19] Berenstein A, Lasjaunias P, ter Brugge KG. Spinal arteriovenous malformations. In: Surgical neuroangiography, clinical and endovascular treatment aspects in adults. Berlin: Springer Verlag 2004;22:738–847.

[20] Berenstein A, Lasjaunias P. Spinal cord arteriovenous malformations. In: Berenstein A, Lasjaunias P, editors, Surgical neuroangiography: endovascular treatment of spine and spinal cord lesions. New York: Springer Verlag 1992;5:24–109.

[21] Kominami S, Liu Y, Alvarez H, et al. A case of VVF presenting with a subarachnoid hemorrhage. Interventional Neuroradiology 1996;2:229–33.

[22] Deans W, Bloch S, Leibrock L, et al. Arteriovenous fistula in patients with neurofibromatosis. Radiology 1982;144:103–7.

[23] Ling JC, Agid R, Nakano S, et al. Metachronous multiplicity of spinal cord arteriovenous fistula and spinal dural AVF in a patient with hereditary hemorrhagic telangiectasia. Interv Neurorad 2005;11:79–86.

[24] Hashimoto T, Wu Y, Lawton MT, et al. Coexpression of angiogenic factors in brain arteriovenous malformations. Neurosurgery 2005;56:1058–65.

[25] Carlson TR, Yan Y, Wu X, et al. Endothelial expression of constitutively active Notch4 elicits reversible arteriovenous malformations in adult mice. Proc Natl Acad Sci U S A 2005;102:9884–9.

[26] Shovlin CL, Guttmacher AE, Buscarini E, et al. Diagnostic criteria for hereditary hemorrhagic telangiectasia (Rendu-Osler-Weber syndrome). Am J Med Genet 2000;91:66–7.

[27] Fernandez-Lopez A, Sanz-Rodriguez F, Blanco FJ, et al. Hereditary hemorrhagic telangiectasia a vascular dysplasia affecting the TGF-B signaling pathway. Clin Med Res 2006;4:66–78.

[28] Begbie ME, Wallace GM, Shovlin CL. Hereditary hemorrhagic telangiectasia (Osler-Weber-Rendu syndrome): a view from the 21st century. Postgrad Med J 2003;79:18–24.

[29] Cole SG, Begbie ME, Wallace GM, et al. A new locus for hereditary haemorrhagic telangiectasia (HHT3) maps to chromosome 5. J Med Genet 2005;42:577–82.

[30] Letteboer TG, Mager HJ, Snijder RJ, et al. J Med Genet 2006;43:371–7.

[31] Marchuk DA, Srinivasan S, Squire TL, et al. Vascular morphogenesis: tales of two syndromes. Hum Mol Genet 2003;12:97–112.

[32] Xu B, Wu YQ, Huey M, et al. Vascular endothelial growth factor induces abnormal microvasculature in the endoglin heterozygous mouse brain. J Cereb Blood Flow Metab 2004;24:237–44.

[33] Pawlikowska L, Tran MN, Achrol AS, et al. Polymorphisms in transforming growth factor-beta related genes in ALK1 and ENG are associated with sporadic brain arteriovenous malformations. Stroke 2005;36:2778.

[34] Krings T, Ozanne A, Chng SM, et al. Neurovascular phenotypes in hereditary hemorrhagic telangiectasia patients according to age. Neuroradiology 2005;47:711–20.

[35] Krings T, Chng SM, Ozanne A, et al. Hereditary hemorrhagic telangiectasia in children: endovascular treatment of neurovascular malformations. Neuroradiology 2005;47:946–54.

[36] Halbach VV, Higashida RT, Dowd CF, et al. Treatment of giant intradural (perimedullary) arteriovenous fistulas. Neurosurgery 1993;33:972–80.

[37] Stephan MJ, Nesbit GM, Behrens ML, et al. Endovascular treatment of spinal arteriovenous fistula in a young child with hereditary hemorrhagic telangiectasia. J Neurosurg 2005;103: 462–5.

[38] Mandzia JL, ter Brugge KG, Faughnan ME, et al. Spinal cord arteriovenous malformations in two patients with hereditary hemorrhagic telangiectasia. Childs Nerv Syst 1999;15:80–3.

[39] Berenbruch K. Ein Fall von multiplen Angiolipomen kombiniert mit einem Angiom des Rueckenmarkes [inaugural dissertation]. Tuebingen (West Germany); 1890. p. 24.

[40] Cobb S. Hemangioma of the spinal cord associated with skin naevi of the same metamere. Ann Surg 1915;62:641–9.

[41] Doppman JL, Wirth FP, Di Chiro G, et al. Value of cutaneous angiomas in the arteriographic localization of spinal-cord arteriovenous malformations. N Engl J Med 1969;281:1140–4.

[42] Matsumaru Y, Pongpech S, Laothamas J, et al. Multifocal and metameric spinal cord arteriovenous malformations. Review of 19 cases. Intervent Neuroradiol 1999;5:27–34.

[43] Soeda A, Sakai N, Lihara K, et al. Cobb syndrome in an infant: treatment with endovascular embolization and corticosteroid therapy: case report. Neurosurgery 2003;52:711–5.

[44] Fukutake T, Kawamura M, Moroo I, et al. [Cobb syndrome and Klippel-Trenaunay-Weber syndrome]. Rinsho Shinkeigaku 1991;31:275–9. [in Japanese].

[45] Pollard SM, Parsons MJ, Kamei M. Essential and overlapping roles for laminin alpha chains in notochord and blood vessel formation. Dev Biol 2006;289:64–76.

[46] Fouquet B, Weinstein BM, Serluca FC, et al. Vessel patterning in the embryo of the zebrafish: guidance by notochord. Dev Biol 1997;183: 37–48.

[47] Alexander MJ, Grossi PM, Spetzler RF, et al. Extradural thoracic arteriovenous malformation in a patient with Klippel-Trenaunay-Weber syndrome. Case report. Neurosurgery 2002;51:1275–8.

[48] Kahara V, Lehto U, Ryymin P, et al. Vertebral epidural arteriovenous fistula and radicular pain in neurofibromatosis type 1. Acta Neurochir (Wien) 2002;144:493–6.

[49] Rodesch G, Alvarez H, Chaskkis C, et al. Clinical manifestations in paraspinal arteriovenous malformations. Spinal cord symptoms, pathophysiology and treatment objectives. Intern J Neuroradiol 1996;2:430–6.

[50] Waitzman AA, Anderson J, Willinsky RA. Endovascular management of vertebral arteriovenous fistulas: the Toronto experience. J Otolaryngol 1996;25:322–8.

[51] Goyal M, Willinsky R, Montanera W, et al. Paravertebral arteriovenous malformations with epidural drainage: clinical spectrum, imaging features, and results of treatment. AJNR Am J Neuroradiol 1999;20:749–55.

[52] Lasjaunias P, Maillot C, ter Brugge K. Pial relations with spinal cord veins explain MRI occult spinal AV shunts. Intervent Neuroradiol 2000; 6:333–6.

[53] Aminoff MJ, Logue V. The prognosis of patients with spinal vascular malformations. Brain 1974;97:211–8.

[54] Krayenbuehl H, Yasargil MG, McClintock HG. Treatment of spinal cord vascular malformations by surgical excision. J Neurosurg 1969;30: 427–35.

[55] Rosenblum B, Oldfield EH, Doppman JL, et al. Spinal arteriovenous malformations: a comparison of dural arteriovenous fistulas and intradural AVMs in 81 patients. J Neurosurg 1987;67: 795–802.

[56] Spetzler RF, Zabramski JM, Flom RA. Management of juvenile spinal AVMs by embolization and surgical excision. J Neurosurg 1989;70: 628–32.

[57] Connolly ES, Zubay GP, McCormick PC, et al. The posterior approach to a series of glomus (type II) intramedullary spinal cord arteriovenous malformations. Neurosurgery 1998;42: 774–86.

[58] Meisel HJ, Mansmann U, Alvarez H, et al. Effect of partial targeted N-butyl-cyano-acrylate embolization in brain AVM. Acta Neurochir (Wien) 2002;144:879–87.

[59] Molyneux AJ, Coley SC. Embolization of spinal cord arteriovenous malformations with an ethylene vinyl alcohol copolymer dissolved in dimethyl sulfoxide (Onyx liquid embolic system). Report of two cases. J Neurosurg 2000; 93(2):304–8.

[60] Niimi Y, Sala F, Deletis V, et al. Neurophysiologic monitoring and pharmacologic provocative testing for embolization of spinal cord arteriovenous malformations. AJNR Am J Neuroradiol 2004;25:1131–8.

[61] Willinsky R, terBrugge K, Montanera W, et al. Spinal epidural arteriovenous fistulas: arterial

and venous approaches to embolization. AJNR Am J Neuroradiol 1993;14:812–7.

[62] Hui F, Trosselo MP, Meisel HJ, et al. Paraspinal arteriovenous shunts in children. Neuroradiology 1994;36:69–73.

[63] Szajner M, Weill A, Piotin M, et al. Endovascular treatment of a cervical paraspinal arteriovenous malformation via arterial and venous approaches. AJNR Am J Neuroradiol 1999;20: 1097–9.

ELSEVIER
SAUNDERS

NEUROIMAGING
CLINICS
OF NORTH AMERICA

Neuroimag Clin N Am 17 (2007) 223–237

Current Endovascular Management of Maxillofacial Vascular Malformations

Yasunari Niimi, MD, PhD*, Joon K. Song, MD,
Alejandro Berenstein, MD

Maxillofacial vascular malformations (MFVMs) are formed due to an error of vascular morphogenesis. They may correspond to a defective remodeling process at the final stages of vessel formation [1]. Although no hereditary MFVMs exist, the defect might be genetically based and secondarily expressed in the first few years of life, such as in Rendu-Osler-Weber syndrome. Vascular malformations generally grow in proportion to the growth of the affected child but may increase in size secondary to various triggering factors such as increased blood flow, arterial occlusion, and venous thrombosis. The development of an individual lesion, especially if it is high flow, may be stimulated by various factors, including endocrine factors (puberty, pregnancy), trauma, iatrogenic insults such as incomplete surgery and proximal embolization, and infection. High flow in an existing MFVM can induce arteriovenous shunting, which, in turn, increases flow demand, cascading enlargement of the malformation. Increased understanding of these additional physiologic variants may help to define their clinical presentation and evolution and assist in designing therapeutic strategies.

Classification and embryogenesis

Vascular malformations are traditionally classified according to the channel abnormalities present and the flow characteristics [2–4]. The various forms of vascular malformations have been considered by some investigators to be caused by arrests occurring at different stages of vascular development. The rarity of fetal diagnosis of vascular malformations except for the lymphatic malformations suggests an embryonic or fetal cellular defect rather than an already abnormal architecturally demonstrable abnormality.

The development of the head and neck area involves complex changes (rotations, invaginations, migrations) of the tissues during the first weeks in the uterus. During normal development of the head and neck, the vasculature undergoes a series of changes in its branching patterns. Regressions

Center for Endovascular Surgery, Institute for Neurology and Neurosurgery, Roosevelt Hospital, 1000 Tenth
Avenue, New York, NY 10019, USA
* Corresponding author.
E-mail address: yniimi@chpnet.org (Y. Niimi).

1052-5149/07/$ – see front matter © 2007 Elsevier Inc. All rights reserved.   doi:10.1016/j.nic.2007.02.002
neuroimaging.theclinics.com

and annexations of arteries account for the unique bidirectional flow in every branch of the head and neck area.

The folds between adjacent buds represent critical areas for capillary maturation, primarily on the venous side. After this has occurred, the arterial system can establish the necessary hemodynamic balance. Delay in bud fusion produces specific arterial anatomic variation. If the maturation of the capillary network is simultaneously delayed, vascular lesions may be seen in association with the arterial variations.

Even if a malformation is present during the development stages, it will remain as a quiescent defect that will be triggered to produce an irreversible fetal, neonatal, child, or adult vascular malformation. Hereditary hemorrhagic telangiectasia produces de novo vascular anomalies over time, often referred to as malformations. The disease gene is recognized to be that for endoglin on chromosome 9q33-34 in some families [5] and activin receptor-like kinase 1 (ACVRL 1) in other families [6]. Families without defects in these two genes have also been reported [7]. The role of growth factors involved in vascular remodeling is probably not restricted to their primary effect; rather, they may serve as multipurpose agents with, for example, a qualitative and quantitative impact on the endothelium (eg, promoters, inhibitors, angiogenetic factors, matrix regulators).

Couly and colleagues [8] demonstrated that endothelial cells of the cephalic region have a regionalized origin from the paraxial mesoderm, which provides blood vessels to specific regions of the face and brain. In general, the neural crest and mesodermal cells originating from a given transverse level occupy the same facial territories, and the two cell types cooperate in myogenesis and in vasculogenesis. Related to this contribution, one can recognize some of the clinical syndromes described in the literature and can postulate a link between apparently unrelated territories. For example, Sturge-Weber syndrome would correspond to a disorder of the rostral mesoderm (medial and lateral) which supplies the prosencephalon and the nasofrontal and maxillary areas. These disorders are collectively called cerebrofacial arteriovenous metameric syndromes [9].

Diagnosis

The diagnosis of an MFVM is usually made based on clinical history and physical examination. A correct history and careful attention to the child's complaints with and without his or her parents present are often sufficient to establish the diagnosis. If the cosmetic aspect is dominant, direct communication

should always be established with the child to temper the demands of the parents.

Cross section noninvasive imaging such as CT or MR imaging is helpful for assessment of the extent of the disease, associated lesions, or multifocality of involvement. MR imaging is the most useful single imaging modality in the investigation of vascular malformations [10] (Fig. 1). The combination of multiplanar spin echo imaging and flow-sensitive sequences permits characterization of the nature and extent of most lesions. CT is less helpful in defining flow characteristics and the extent of vascular malformations but is useful in demonstrating the nature and extent of bony involvement and the presence of phleboliths, which are pathognomonic of venous malformations. Ultrasound, including Doppler techniques, is a modality for determining tissue and flow characteristics in superficial lesions but is suboptimal in demonstrating the extent of lesions. Plain radiographs are useful in selected patients, mainly to document bony changes. For example, a simple panoramic (Panorex) radiograph may suffice to follow the bony changes in dental arteriovenous malformations. Angiography is reserved for patients in whom a decision has been made to intervene and is generally performed at the same time as embolization. Exceptionally, angiography may be necessary to confirm the diagnosis and to demonstrate the extent of the soft tissue capillary or arteriovenous malformations or fistulas. The advent of three-dimensional rotational angiography is expanding our ability to study intraosseous arteriovenous malformations.

Treatment goal and strategy

MFVMs are challenging to treat and require the skills of multiple disciplines. Management of these lesions is best achieved by a specialist who understands the various clinical expressions of the problem, the natural history of the lesion, and the needs of the child. Such a specialist diagnoses the lesion, establishes clinical and morphologic objectives, and then introduces the problem to other specialists for management strategies. Over the last 10 years, the advancement of surgical techniques aided by preoperative, intraoperative, or postoperative embolization has created a new group of specialists combining competence in endovascular, plastic and reconstructive head and neck, and maxillofacial surgery in children [11–18].

Because they are usually nonlethal lesions, the primary goal of treatment is to restore and preserve function, stop and control bleeding, and improve or restore cosmesis. Partial treatment in a less risky and less invasive method may be more beneficial to

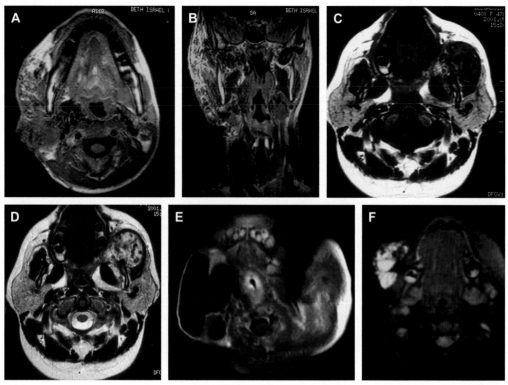

Fig. 1. (*A, B*) T1-weighted axial (*A*) and coronal (*B*) MR images of a right soft tissue arteriovenous malformation involving the parotid space, malar soft tissue including the masseter muscle extending superficially to the sub-cutaneous fat and deep adjacent to the oropharynx. Heterogeneous signals including flow voids are seen. (*C, D*) T1-weighted MR image with contrast (*C*) and T2-weighted (*D*) axial image of a venous vascular malformation involving the left masseter muscle with a small component in the masticator space. Round signal voids indicate the existence of phleboliths typical for venous vascular malformations. (*E, F*) T1-weighted axial MR image with contrast (*E*) and T2 fat suppression (*F*) image of a macrocystic lymphatic malformation. Multiple cysts with different protein densities are seen superficial and deep to the sternocleidomastoid muscle and superior malar soft tissue. Fluid-fluid levels are seen in the upper portion (*F*).

the patient than aggressive curative treatment. MFVMs in children under 10 years of age may interfere with natural growth and maturation of the maxillomandibular frame, causing malocclusion of the mouth or modeling defects owing to external pressure on the forming bones or sinuses. Early intervention can arrest or even reverse such changes. The main indications for early management of vascular malformations are as follows:

Dental arcade stabilization
Osseous remodeling
Recurrent hemorrhagic complications
Mass effect (swallowing, growing)
Episodic swelling and airway compromise
Neurologic impairment

Several questions should be answered to set up an appropriate treatment goal for a child with an MFVM: (1) the nature of the malformation, (2) the type and extent of existing damage, (3) the potential future development of the lesion, (4) the

ability to arrest the progression of the disease and to restore damaged function, and (5) the future availability of newly developing treatment techniques.

Specific problems and treatment in each subcategory of MFVM are discussed in the following sections.

Arteriovenous Shunts

An arteriovenous malformation consists of a nidus or network of abnormal vascular channels with feeding arteries and draining veins. Except for extremely rare high-flow lesions, which may present with cardiac overload in neonates and infants, most soft tissue arteriovenous malformations are asymptomatic in the first 1 to 2 decades of life. They often manifest as a cutaneous blush with or without underlying soft tissue hypertrophy. Clinical findings include local hyperthermia, prominent pulsations, thrill, and bruit. Development of these lesions often seems to be precipitated by hormonal factors (puberty, pregnancy, and hormone therapy), trauma, infection, or iatrogenic causes (surgery, embolization). Close follow-up is essential for an arteriovenous malformation because it may extend, especially after incomplete surgical intervention or proximal embolization, into surrounding tissues or territories that initially did not appear to be involved. Venous hypertension results in tissue ischemia, ultimately leading to pain and skin ulceration, often associated with severe bleeding.

If complete eradication cannot be obtained with combined approaches for symptomatic arteriovenous malformations, the authors recommend partial, targeted endovascular embolization with a liquid agent to control the lesion. Surgical partial treatment often triggers expansion of the arteriovenous lesions and should be avoided unless life-threatening bleeding cannot be controlled by transarterial or direct percutaneous embolization. In many cases, the subsequent increase of the abnormal network of vessels after partial surgical resection of the lesion is difficult to treat because it involves normal reactive vascularization. Any attempt at this stage to improve the appearance may lead to tissue ischemia. The authors also try to delay major facial surgical reconstructions involving the skeleton before the completion of maxillofacial growth.

Soft tissue arteriovenous malformations

Arteriovenous malformations can involve the soft tissues in various extensions.

Intramuscular arteriovenous malformations Intramuscular arteriovenous malformations may be associated with pain (eg, trismus). These arteriovenous lesions are rarely strictly limited to a single muscle; when they are, they usually involve a masticator muscle. They are seldom of the arteriovenous type but are rather venous lesions. Some lesions are small and clinically difficult to demonstrate; they appear as recurrent hematomas, particularly in the masseteric muscle where lysed hematoma may be diagnosed as a cystic lesion. Surgical exploration of these lesions demonstrates small malformations on the wall of the cavity.

Cutaneous arteriovenous malformations Cutaneous arteriovenous malformations initially demonstrate a superficial blush discoloration and warmth (Fig. 2). As they develop, the color intensifies and tortuous, tense veins appear. Dystrophic changes, ulceration, bleeding, and persistent pain may follow. MR imaging confirms the diagnosis of an arteriovenous malformation and demonstrates its extent, although it is often difficult to distinguish between the actual nidus and the feeding and draining vessels. Trauma is a frequent cause of

the growth of the lesion, with hemorrhagic complications, particularly in children and external ear arteriovenous malformations. With clinical examination, midline located arteriovenous fistulas of the forehead can easily be differentiated from sinus pericranii. Associated abnormalities are exceptional, and investigations of the intracranial structures depend on the degree of suspicion.

Treatment must be planned carefully to avoid stimulating progression and interfering with future management. Surgical ligation or endovascular occlusion of proximal feeding vessels must be avoided [14]. Superselective targeted arterial embolization is indicated to decrease symptoms such as pain, bleeding, and ischemic ulceration [3,14,19]. Embolization should be performed with permanent agents such as tissue adhesive whenever possible. High-flow cervicofacial arteriovenous malformations are difficult to exclude by arterial embolization alone and should be treated in combination with embolization and surgery. Single-hole arteriovenous fistulas can be easily treated by transarterial embolization. Lesions that are amenable to complete excision are best treated by presurgical embolization and excision [11,13,20]. Large lesions involving the skin surface may be well treated with extensive excision and microvascular soft tissue grafting prepared with a tissue expander [21]. Conservative treatment should also be considered for certain lesions.

Intraosseous arteriovenous malformations

Intraosseous arteriovenous malformations are rare and have been overdiagnosed. In most instances, the misdiagnosis results from an erroneous interpretation of bony changes associated with a soft tissue arteriovenous malformation. Soft tissue arteriovenous malformations are often associated with bony defects owing to compression by dilated draining veins. Bony hypertrophy is also seen as a consequence of venous and lymphatic interference related to an adjacent soft tissue arteriovenous malformation. These secondary changes must be distinguished from truly intraosseous arteriovenous malformations.

Mandibular and maxillary arteriovenous malformations Patients with a maxillary or mandibular arteriovenous malformation often present with life-threatening hemorrhage related to tooth eruption, dental infection, and dental extraction (Fig. 3). This malformation can be managed by arterial embolization followed by extraction of involved teeth [12,13]. Bone erosion surrounding teeth may be best shown with CT or panoramic radiography. In the authors' experience, arterial embolization combined with direct injection of

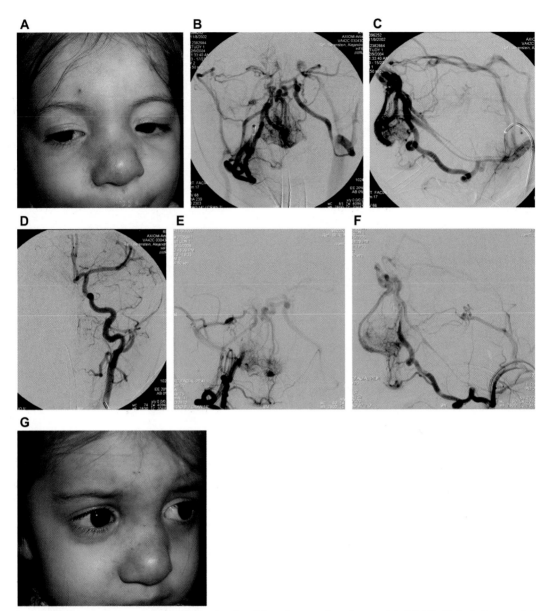

Fig. 2. Soft tissue arteriovenous malformation involving the nose in a 2-year-old girl. (*A*) Clinical picture of the patient before treatment showing reddish discoloration and swelling of the nose and forehead. (*B, C*) Right facial artery angiogram in posteroanterior (PA) (*B*) and lateral (*C*) projections showing arteriovenous malformation involving the nose. (*D*) Left common carotid artery angiogram in PA projection showing a small contribution to the nose arteriovenous malformation from the left external carotid artery branches. (*E, F*) Right facial artery angiogram in PA and lateral projections after endovascular embolization showing significantly decreased vascularity of the nose arteriovenous malformation. (*G*) Clinical picture after embolization showing improvement of discoloration and swelling.

tissue adhesive into the intramandibular nidus and draining vein can achieve stable hemostasis and even complete exclusion of the nidus with reossification of the affected mandible. This approach is preferred to mandibulectomy, especially in the immature facial skeleton [13,22,23]. Proximal vessel ligation or embolization should be avoided because it leads to recruitment of collateral supply to the lesion and induces nonsprouting angiogenesis indistinguishable from the nidus, which makes subsequent treatment more difficult.

The authors analyzed the long-term experience in 31 patients with vascular malformations involving the maxilla and mandible who were treated

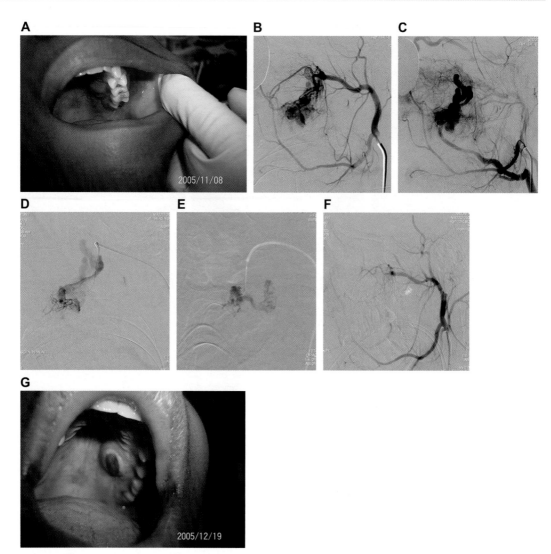

Fig. 3. Maxillary arteriovenous malformation in a 12-year-old male patient with several episodes of severe hemorrhage from the gingiva. (*A*) Clinical picture before treatment showing a soft tissue pulsatile mass in the left gingiva and palate. (*B, C*) Early (*B*) and late (*C*) phases of the left external carotid artery angiogram in the lateral projection showing a left maxillary arteriovenous malformation with large draining venous channel inside the maxilla. (*D*) Lateral view of the superselective angiogram of the left descending palatine artery showing arteriovenous shunts to the intraosseous vein. (*E*) N-butyl cyanoacrylate (NBCA) cast injected from the same microcatheter position as in (*D*), showing penetration of NBCA into the vein. (*F*) Lateral view of the external carotid artery angiogram after multiple embolization showing disappearance of the arteriovenous malformation. (*G*) Clinical picture after embolization showing ulceration of the left palate. No further hemorrhagic episodes were experienced.

primarily with endovascular therapy from 1979 to 2001 [13]. All of the patients underwent embolization as definitive treatment, palliative therapy, or preoperatively for a planned surgical resection. The group consisted of 13 males and 18 females with a mean age of 16 years at initial presentation (range, 1–55 years). The average duration of follow-up was 6.7 years (range, 1–22 years). Thirteen patients had mandibular involvement, 13 had maxillary involvement, and five had combined maxilla and mandible

malformations. There were 26 (84%) arterial, four (12%) venous, and one (4%) capillary malformations. Adjacent soft tissues were involved to various degrees. This involvement was more significant in maxillar lesions than in mandibular lesions. Twenty-eight patients (90%) had bleeding, and all of the patients with mandibular or combined maxillary/mandibular vascular malformations presented with this symptom. Most bleeding originated from the gingival or alveolar ridge and was spontaneous with dental eruption or associated with loose teeth. The second most common cause of bleeding was iatrogenic from attempted biopsy, mass excision, or dental extraction. Epistaxis was a common presenting symptom with maxillary vascular malformations. Facial asymmetry and swelling occurred in 61% of patients, followed by pain in 35%.

Six females (33%) experienced exacerbation of their symptoms with hormonal changes during their menstrual cycle or pregnancy. One patient had no evidence of a vascular malformation until pregnancy when swelling and subsequent oral bleeding started. Two patients with arterial vascular malformations of the maxilla/mandible with extensive soft tissue involvement experienced high-output cardiac failure.

Based on the authors' experience, embolization is the treatment of choice and was the only treatment in 81% of cases [13]. In 19% of patients, embolization was followed by surgery. Bleeding symptoms were controlled in all patients, and no patients had progression of disease. Among patients with mandibular lesions regardless of the type of malformation, nine patients (70%) were cured, two patients (15%) improved, and two patients (15%) were stable. All of the patients with a mandibular malformation without soft tissue involvement were cured. A lower cure rate of 46% was obtained for six patients who had maxillary vascular malformations, and none of the patients with combined mandibular/maxillary malformations were cured of their disease, although four of these patients (80%) had stabilization of the lesions. Overall, 15 patients (48%) were cured, five patients (16%) had improvement, and 11 patients (35%) had stable lesions. In the continuing care of these patients, 11 patients had dental extractions combined with embolization to prevent severe hemorrhage. One drawback of acrylic embolization in this area was the development of local foreign body reaction to the embolic material, which required multiple debridements for sequestered bone or infection from retained foreign body embolic material. Laser treatment for cutaneous manifestations of vascular malformations in three patients resulted in improved cosmesis.

Thirteen patients had temporary treatment complications, including ischemic ulceration/necrosis in seven patients, osteomyelitis/infection in seven patients, and temporary visual disturbance in three patients. Temporary numbness along the inferior alveolar nerve distribution, transient facial nerve paralysis, pulmonary embolism from dislodgement of embolic material, and the development of a cataract from radiation were additional complications, all successfully treated without further consequences.

Embolization of facial arteriovenous malformations can be performed even after proximal ligation or embolization by direct puncture of the feeding arteries or nidus, arterial cut-down, or surgical arterial reconstruction [14].

Intraosseous slow-flow malformations A rare group of intraosseous vascular malformations present with expansion of the bony cortex, presenting as a nonpainful mass with bony changes of expansion suggestive of an aggressive behavior (Fig. 4). The authors have seen three such cases. Usually, an attempt at biopsy is associated with bleeding. Angiography fails to show vascularity in the arterial or capillary phase but may show some pooling of contrast material in the late phase. All cases have responded to direct alcohol sclerotherapy with reossification.

Arteriolar-capillary malformations

Arteriolar-capillary malformations constitute a rare subgroup of vascular lesions that are currently recognized as noninvoluting capillary hemangiomas [24]. These lesions are described in the article on hemangiomas by Song and colleagues in this issue.

Capillary venous malformations

Capillary venous malformations include port-wine stains and telangiectasias [25,26] and usually involve the skin surface. They are usually sporadic, but families with a dominant inheritance pattern with incomplete penetrance have been reported. Linkage analysis has identified a locus on chromosome 5q13-15 (CMC1) [27,28]. The causative gene for CMC1 was identified as a negative regulator of Ras and was called p120-RasGAP or *RASA1* [29]. Some affected members have more complex vascular malformations comprising capillary venous malformations and arteriovenous malformations, such as in Parkes Weber, Sturge-Weber, or Klippel-Trenaunay syndromes [29]. Port-wine stains are often associated with progressive thickening of the skin and subcutaneous layers as well as overgrowth of the underlying facial skeleton, often resulting in facial asymmetry and dental malalignment. These port-wine stains almost always present in infancy. The shape and the link with the trigeminal nerve territory are of no clinical importance. Approximately 1% to 2% of patients with port-wine stains have Sturge-Weber syndrome. The intracranial manifestations are generally not present in patients with port-wine stains confined to V2 and V3. CT and MR imaging findings may be absent in the first 1 to 2 years of life. Facial capillary venous malformations may include subjacent lymphatic malformations. In this case, bone deformity is demonstrated, particularly of the maxilla.

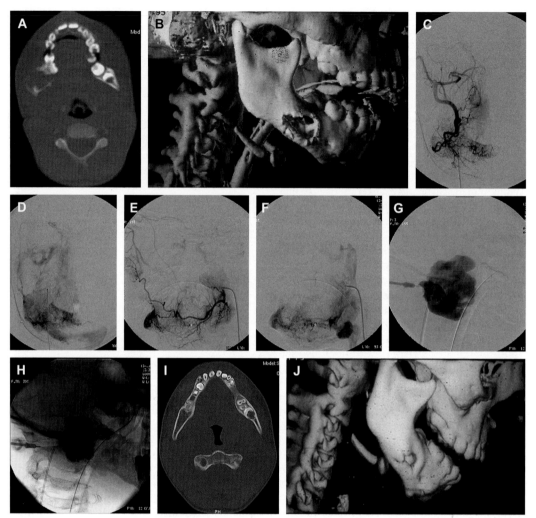

Fig. 4. Intraosseous slow-flow malformation in a 7-year-old male presenting with a nonpainful, nonpulsatile right mandibular mass. Blood was obtained by needle biopsy of the lesion. (*A, B*) Axial CT (*A*) and three-dimensional reconstruction of the bone (*B*) demonstrating an expansile destruction of the body of the mandible. (*C–F*) Early (*C, E*) and late (*D, F*) phases of the PA (*C, D*) and lateral (*E, F*) views of the right facial artery angiogram showing a slow filling of the venous pouch with stagnation of the contrast. (*G, H*) Direct puncture contrast injection in oblique view with (*G*) and without (*H*) subtraction, showing accumulation of contrast material in the venous pouch. This area was treated with direct ethanol injection. (*I, J*) Axial CT (*I*) and three-dimensional reconstruction of the bone (*J*) 2 years after treatment showing reossification and healing of the bone destruction.

Telangiectasias are also primarily venous lesions, but they are exceptional in children. The remodeling process is impaired because of an abnormal binding protein (endoglin) which compromises locally the normal reconstitution of the venous capillary junction.

There is almost no indication for embolization in these types of lesions. When reconstruction of a hyperemic facial skeleton is considered, presurgical embolization with particles should be considered to reduce surgical blood loss.

Venous vascular malformations

These lesions are the most frequent vascular malformation. The lesions are typically nonpulsatile, soft and compressible, distend with Valsalva maneuvers, are easily emptied by manual compression, and are frequently multifocal and bilateral. Overexpression of the Tie-2 gene on chromosome 9p was identified in two multiple cutaneous and mucosal venous malformation families [30–32]. Development of abnormal vessels in this syndrome is caused by a local uncoupling of endothelial smooth muscle cell signaling [30]. Some families do not show linkage to the Tie-2 locus, suggesting the existence of additional loci for inherited venous vascular malformations. The skin temperature over the lesion is normal. The lesions have variable clinical presentations depending on their depth and extent [26,33]. When superficial, they are characterized by a bluish discoloration of the skin or mucosa. They can be discreet or can become disfiguring and may compromise the airway or the swallowing pathway. When they are located in deeper planes, there may be no discoloration, and the lesion may present as a fluctuating mass that increases in size with the Valsalva maneuver, changes of position, or mastication when it involves the muscles of mastication.

Most of these lesions consist of spongy masses of sinusoidal spaces and have variable communications with adjacent veins. Alternatively, some venous malformations represent varicosities or dysplasias of small and large venous channels [34,35]. They typically contain phleboliths, which are pathognomonic if present.

Characteristic MR imaging findings include focal or diffuse collections of high T2 signal, often containing identifiable spaces of variable size separated by septations [3]. Phleboliths may be evident as areas of signal void, which are most prominent on gradient echo images. Flow-sensitive images demonstrate no high-flow vessels within or around the lesions but may show evidence of old thrombus. Contrast administration results in variable enhancement ranging from dense enhancement similar to that in adjacent veins to non-homogeneous or delayed enhancement. CT imaging likewise shows variable contrast enhancement with or without rounded lamellate calcifications. Angiography is not necessary to make the diagnosis but typically shows either no filling of the malformation or delayed opacification of sinusoidal spaces with a grape-like appearance with or without dysplastic draining veins when using a long contrast injection [2]. Direct percutaneous catheterization of the malformation with contrast injection shows the interconnecting sinusoidal spaces. Careful attention should be paid to the communication between the drainage and transcranial, orbital, or vertebral venous channels.

Direct injection of a sclerosing agent, including 98% ethanol, sodium tetradecyl sulfate, sodium morrhuate, or sodium ducal, results in thrombosis and gradual shrinkage of the malformation and is the preferred treatment [34,36–39] (Fig. 5). The authors have no experience with other agents, including prolamine and polidocanol [40].

The technique of sclerotherapy involves percutaneous catheterization of the malformation using a needle or Teflon-sheathed needle cannula. After confirming free blood return, contrast is injected, recording with serial angiographic imaging or under the live-subtraction mode to document the cannula position within the malformation and the presence or absence of venous outflow. In the presence of significant venous outflow, local compression over the venous outflow is applied during injection of sclerosing agents. If there is drainage toward the intracranial venous system where compression is not possible, liquid coils can be placed to block the undesired drainage.

The most common complication of ethanol sclerotherapy is skin or mucous necrosis and neuropathy. Skin blistering or full-thickness necrosis is likely to occur if the malformation involves the skin or mucosal surface. The authors use facial nerve monitoring to avoid facial nerve damage. The total volume of injected ethanol should not exceed 0.3 mL/kg in children below the age of 2 years and 0.6 mL/kg in older children. One should prevent alcohol from escaping into the systemic circulation because it may produce severe pulmonary vasoconstriction that can be fatal. Cardiac dysrhythmias can also occur related to overinjection of alcohol, including bradycardia, arrhythmias, and cardiac arrest. Treatment of large malformations is usually staged to avoid complications related to the amount of sclerosing agents.

Recanalization after sclerotherapy depends on the single versus multicompartmental nature of the lesion. A single cavity is likely to be excluded in one treatment, whereas multiple cavity or previously operated malformations require multiple punctures and tend to result in incomplete occlusion. In the event of recurrence following sclerotherapy, surgical resection should be considered if feasible. In general, the more localized deep venous malformations and small cutaneous or mucosal lesions respond well to direct injection of the sclerosing agent. Diffuse lesions are more resistant to treatment. Venous malformations of the tongue and airway can often be treated successfully with sclerotherapy following tracheostomy, although laser photocoagulation has recently been proven to be effective [41]. For extensive cervicofacial venous malformations, staged sclerotherapy can have a dramatic effect in reducing size and improving appearance over time.

In very young children, venous vascular malformations may remodel maxillofacial bones. Early intervention is indicated in such cases to reverse these changes.

More recently, the authors have increasingly performed surgical excision of venous vascular malformations 24 to 36 hours after sclerotherapy in well-defined lesions, taking advantage of the

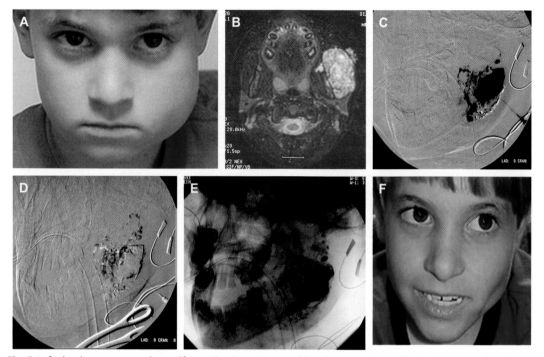

Fig. 5. Left cheek venous vascular malformation in an 8-year-old male presenting with cheek asymmetry. The left cheek increased in size by Valsalva maneuver. (A) Clinical picture before treatment showing left cheek mass. (B) T2-weighted, fat-saturated axial MR image showing a mass with heterogeneous signal intensity in the left masseter muscle extending to the masticator space. (C) Injection of 75% ethanol mixed with Ethiodol under live subtraction mode showing accumulation of the sclerosing agent in the lesion. (D) Further injection of the sclerosing agent with compression of the venous outflow of the lesion. (E) Non-subtracted image of the head after sclerotherapy showing stasis of the sclerosing agent within the lesion. (F) Clinical picture 5 months after treatment showing decreased size of the left cheek mass.

thrombosed malformation and the surrounding edema that facilitates developing a surgical plane of demarcation between the malformation and normal tissue (Waner Berenstein, unpublished data, 2006) (Fig. 6).

Lymphatic malformations

Lymphatic malformations may be classified as macrocystic or microcystic. Those in the head and neck result from maldevelopment of the cervicofacial lymphatic system, which normally begins as paired jugular lymph sacs sprouting from the primitive jugular venous plexus in the 6-week-old embryo [42]. The jugular sacs and channels normally spread to connect with the subclavian (axillary) lymph sacs, which then extend caudally, anastomosing with the internal thoracic, paratracheal, and thoracic ducts. Extensions of the jugular sac channels ultimately communicate with lymphatic channels of the head, neck, and upper limb that have sprouted from peripheral veins. The macrocystic types of lymphatic malformations (cystic hygromas) are thought to result from maldevelopment of the primitive jugular subclavian and axillary sacs, possibly by failure to re-establish venous connections. Interruption or obstruction of the peripheral lymphatic channels presumably results in diffuse or microcystic lymphatic malformations (ie, lymphangiomas).

Lymphatic malformations are usually evident at birth. Macrocystic lesions are most commonly located in the neck, axilla, and chest wall and may be massive and interfere with the birth process. Microcystic lesions usually present as diffuse soft tissue thickening, often associated with an overlying capillary malformation or vesicles of the skin or mucosa. The lesions typically grow proportionally with the child but undergo episodic swelling, often associated with signs of inflammation, either spontaneously or in association with regional infections. Acute enlargement may be related to lymphatic obstruction or hemorrhage. Communications between the macrocystic lymphatic malformations and adjacent veins are frequently present. On physical examination, lymphatic malformations have a rubbery or cystic consistency. Typically, they cannot be manually decompressed like venous malformations.

MR imaging findings in macrocystic lymphatic malformations include cystic fluid collections,

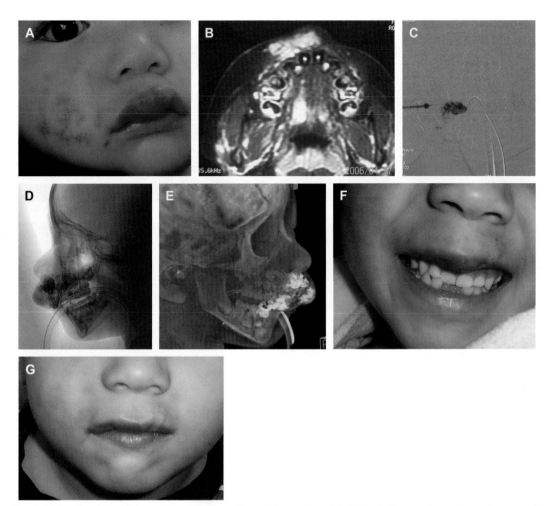

Fig. 6. Right cheek and upper lip venous vascular malformation. (*A*) Clinical picture when the patient was 10 months old, showing discoloration and swelling of the upper lip and anterior cheek. (*B*) T1-weighted, fat-saturated axial MR image with contrast showing the upper lip and the right palate lesions. (*C*) Direct puncture contrast injection to the upper lip lesion under subtraction mode. (*D*) Non-subtracted lateral view of the face after injection of 75% ethanol mixed with Ethiodol showing radiopaque sclerosing agent in the upper lip lesion. (*E*) Three-dimensional reconstructed bone image showing radiopaque sclerosing agent in the upper lip lesion. (*F*) Clinical picture when the patient was 6 years old after three sessions of sclerosing therapy, showing decreased size of the upper lip lesion. (*G*) Clinical picture when the patient was 6 years old after surgical resection of the upper lip lesion, showing further improvement of the appearance.

often with fluid-fluid levels, associated with a rim of no contrast enhancement. Evidence of hemorrhage or thrombosis may be present. Enlargement of adjacent veins, including the jugular, paravertebral, and superior vena cava, has been described in cervicofacial lymphatic malformations [43,44]. Microcystic lymphatic malformations typically appear as diffuse "sheets" of bright signal on T2-weighted spin echo MR imaging, usually with various contrast enhancement patterns. The adjacent subcutaneous fat often shows evidence of lymphedema. CT best demonstrates the bone distortion and shows the soft tissue component of the malformation to be of lower density than surrounding muscle.

Treatment of macrocystic lymphatic malformations is generally staged early surgical excision. In selected cases of extensive lesions, sclerotherapy may be successful. Residual or recurrent cysts after surgery may also be treated by injection of sclerosing agents. A wide range of sclerosing drugs have been used in the past with variable results. The most recent sclerosing agent reported to be effective in some lymphatic malformations is deoxycylcline, OK-432 (Picibanil), a derivative of the streptococcal bacterium, which has been used to induce inflammation and subsequent fibrosis [45–47]. The authors have had long lasting effects with ethanol sclerotherapy in macrocystic cases (Figs. 7 and 8).

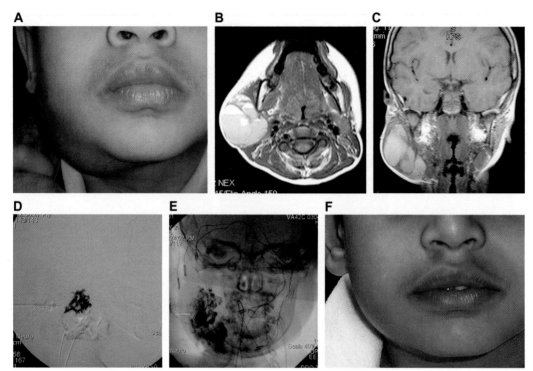

Fig. 7. Right retromandibular macrocystic lymphatic malformation in a 4-year-old boy. (*A*) Clinical picture before treatment showing retromandibular mass. (*B, C*) T1-weighted axial (*B*) and coronal (*C*) MR images showing a multicystic lesion with different signal intensities posterior to the mandible. (*D*) Subtracted image of direct puncture contrast injection in the lateral view showing accumulation of contrast material without venous drainage. (*E*) Non-subtracted image of the face after sclerotherapy with 75% ethanol mixed with Ethiodol showing radiopaque sclerosing agent in the lesion. (*F*) Clinical picture after two sessions of treatment showing decreased size of the retromandibular mass.

More recently, the addition of laser photocoagulation has further improved the treatment results of conjunctival lesions.

Sclerotherapy is performed in a similar fashion to the treatment of venous malformations. The cystic spaces in lymphatic malformations often do not interconnect, making sclerotherapy less effective. In larger compartments, a yellowish or serosanguinous fluid can be collected, and a similar volume of ethanol is injected. Microcystic lymphatic malformations are difficult to treat by any means owing to their diffuse nature and infiltration of the tissue layers. The role of sclerotherapy is limited to symptomatic areas of repeated swelling and bleeding.

An important part of the overall management of these children is the need for long-term prophylactic antibiotic therapy to prevent or ameliorate the repeated infections. Antibiotics with a broad or medium spectrum are rotated every 3 to 4 weeks to avoid the development of resistance.

Venolymphatic malformations (hematolymphangiomas) are often located in the tongue, where they provoke macroglossia. The lymphatic character is established by acute swelling with infection, their usual regression, and the residual mucous vesicles. The venous character is expressed by the dark, often black color of the tongue during the crisis and the slightly hemorrhagic aspect of the dry tongue permanently protracted during the swelling episodes. To avoid the open bite syndrome and difficult mandibular growth, early embolization is recommended. In the authors' experience, the response of such tongue lesions to transarterial embolization with particles has been excellent, with a decrease in the frequency and intensity of swelling or even disappearance. Orthodontic treatment can correct most open bite syndromes resulting from the permanent macroglossia. In some instances, cuneiform glossectomy has been performed following embolization to allow the tongue to remain behind the teeth.

Mixed vascular malformations

Mixed vascular malformations are common. Particularly, capillary malformations of the skin are often present in association with a deep arteriovenous malformation or deep lymphatic or venous malformations. Another common combination is that of

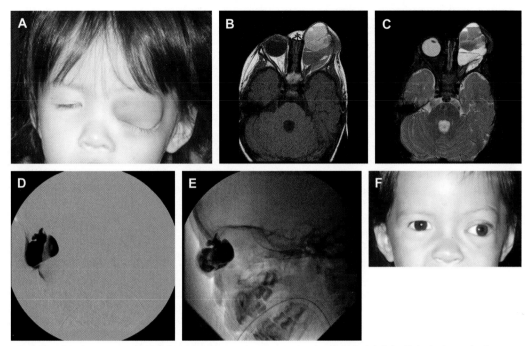

Fig. 8. Left orbital macrocystic lymphatic malformation in an 18-month-old girl. (*A*) Clinical picture before treatment showing discoloration and swelling of the left eye lid. (*B, C*) T1- (*B*) and T2-weighted (*C*) axial MR images showing a multicystic lesion in the left orbit with different signal intensities and fluid-fluid levels, typical for lymphatic malformation. No extension to the orbital apex. (*D*) Subtracted lateral view of direct puncture contrast injection to the lesion showing accumulation of the contrast without venous drainage. (*E*) Non-subtracted image of the face in the lateral view after treatment with ethanol and sodium morrhuate, showing radiopaque sclerosing agent in the lesion. (*F*) Clinical picture 6 months after treatment showing decreased size of the lesion and improvement of the appearance.

combined lymphatic and venous malformations. The lymphatic and venous systems develop very closely in time, and it is not unexpected that malformations of both systems will coexist. A diffuse lymphatic malformation is often associated with varicosities of adjacent draining veins. In particular, lymphatic malformations of the head and neck are frequently associated with markedly dilated brachiocephalic veins or the superior vena cava. In addition, dysplastic venous channels may coexist with lymphatic malformations, and hemorrhage into lymphatic cysts is assumed to be caused by communications between the lymphatic system and veins.

False maxillofacial vascular malformations

Vascular malformations should be differentiated from vascular anomalies and from facial venous dilatations which can be idiopathic or secondary to intracranial vascular lesions.

Idiopathic facial vascular (venous) dilatations

Parents and pediatricians are sometimes concerned about prominent veins in infants and young children. Auscultation of the head increases this anxiety if it reveals a cranial bruit. Such pulsatile bruit is usually benign and regresses spontaneously. Its frequency is increased up to the age of 3 years and then diminishes. These bruits are rare in neonates. They are most likely due to blood turbulences in the veins of the skull base. The growing skull base can rapidly adapt to the hemodynamic venous conditions of the walking child. These dilated facial veins indicate the early opening of the brain venous outlets into the cavernous sinus.

When confronted with dilated frontal facial veins associated with an intracranial bruit, one needs to exclude the possibility of an early manifestation of an intracranial arteriovenous shunt. CT imaging of the brain without and with contrast administration is usually enough to eliminate an arteriovenous shunt or a unilateral dural sinus occlusion. The authors have not encountered any arteriovenous malformation revealed only by an intracranial bruit in the pediatric population in the presence of normal CT. Clinical follow-up is mandatory to confirm the spontaneous disappearance of the veins and the bruit before the age of 7 years. If CT is abnormal, diagnostic angiography should be performed to outline the abnormality.

Facial venous dilatation associated with intracranial vascular lesions

Facial veins can provide evidence of important hemodynamic intracranial disorders in which the venous blood is re-routed toward the cavernous sinus. During infancy, this becomes a possible outlet for cerebral venous drainage, and the orbit is then an alternative communication passage between the endocranium and the facial veins via the superior ophthalmic vein. Two different situations are associated with transorbital drainage: (1) the brain drains through the orbit, while the intracranial arteriovenous shunt drains separately into the posterior sinuses; or (2) the jugular foramen is occluded, and both the lesion and the brain compete to drain through the orbit, but often also transcranially across the vault. In the former situation, the neurocognitive prognosis is excellent because the brain does not suffer the consequences of the shunt; conversely, in the latter situation, the neurologic prognosis is poor, and early management is required to avoid seizures, deficits, or hemorrhagic episodes.

Regression of these facial veins can only be obtained once the treatment is completed. In some instances, regression is not complete, particularly if the posterior outlets are no longer patent and if the communications across the skull base are insufficient.

References

[1] Folkman J, D'Amore PA. Blood vessel formation: what is its molecular basis? Cell 1996;87:1153–5.

[2] Burrows PE, Mulliken JB, Fellows KE, et al. Childhood hemangiomas and vascular malformations: angiographic differentiation. AJR Am J Roentgenol 1983;141:483–8.

[3] Jackson IT, Carreno R, Potparic Z, et al. Hemangiomas, vascular malformations, and lymphovenous malformations: classification and methods of treatment. Plast Reconstr Surg 1993;91:1216–30.

[4] Mulliken JB, Glowacki J. Hemangiomas and vascular malformations in infants and children: a classification based on endothelial characteristics. Plast Reconstr Surg 1982;69:412–22.

[5] McAllister KA, Grogg KM, Johnson DW, et al. Endoglin, a TGF-β binding protein of endothelial cells, is the gene for hereditary haemorrhagic telangiectasias type 1. Nat Genet 1994;8:345–51.

[6] Johnson DW, Berg JN, Baldwin MA, et al. Mutations in the activin receptor-like kinase 1 gene in hereditary haemorrhagic telangiectasias type 2. Nat Genet 1996;13:441–3.

[7] Piantanida M, Buscarini E, Dellavecchia C, et al. Hereditary haemorrhagic telangiectasia with extensive liver involvement is not caused by either HHT1 or HHT2. J Med Genet 1996;33:441–3.

[8] Couly G, Coltey P, Eichmann A, et al. The angiogenetic potentials of the cephalic mesoderm and the origin of brain and head blood vessels. Mech Dev 1995;53:97–112.

[9] Bhattachaya JJ, Luo CB, Suh DC. Wyburn-Mason or Bonnet-Dechume-Blanc as cerebrofacial arteriovenous metameric syndromes (CAMS): a new concept and new classification. Interventional Neuroradiology 2001;7(1):5–17.

[10] Yuh WT, Buehner LS, Kao SC, et al. Magnetic resonance imaging of pediatric head and neck cystic hygromas. Ann Otol Rhinol Laryngol 1991;100:737–42.

[11] Berenstein A, Scott J, Choi IS, et al. Percutaneous embolization of the arteriovenous fistulas of the external carotid artery. AJNR Am J Neuroradiol 1986;7:937–42.

[12] Persky M, Berenstein A. Management of vascular lesions of the nose and paranasal sinuses. In: Goldman J, editor. The principles and practice of rhinology. New York: Churchill Livingstone; 1987. p. 569–80.

[13] Persky MS, Yoo HJ, Berenstein A. Management of vascular malformations of the mandible and maxilla. Laryngoscope 2003;113:1885–92.

[14] Riles TS, Berenstein A, Fisher FS, et al. Reconstruction of the ligated external carotid artery for embolization of cervicofacial arteriovenous malformations. J Vasc Surg 1993;17:491–8.

[15] Waner M, Suen JY. Treatment options for the management of hemangiomas. In: Waner M, Suen JY, editors. Hemangiomas and vascular malformations of the head and neck. New York: Wiley-Liss; 1999. p. 233–61.

[16] Seccia A, Sakarello M, Farallo E, et al. Combined radiologic and surgical treatment of arteriovenous malformations of the head and neck. Ann Plast Surg 1999;43:359–66.

[17] Hubbell RN, Ihm PS. Current surgical management of vascular anomalies. Curr Opin Otolaryngol Head Neck Surg 2000;8(6):441–7.

[18] Lee BB, Bergan JJ. Advanced management of congenital vascular malformations: a multidisciplinary approach. Cardiovasc Surg 2002;10(6):523–33.

[19] Burrows PE, Lasjaunias PL, Ter Brugge KG, et al. Urgent and emergent embolization of lesions of the head and neck in children: indication and results. Pediatrics 1987;80:386–94.

[20] Goldberg RA, Garcia GH, Duckwiler GR. Combined embolization and surgical treatment of arteriovenous malformation of the orbit. Am J Opthalmol 1993;116:17–25.

[21] Marotta TR, Berenstein A, Zide B. The combined role of embolization and tissue expander in the management of arteriovenous malformations of the scalp. Am J Neuroradiol 1994;15:1240–6.

[22] Chiras J, Hassine D, Goudot P, et al. Treatment of arteriovenous malformations of the mandible by arterial and venous embolization. AJNR Am J Neuroradiol 1990;11:1191–4.

[23] Shultz RE, Richardson DD, Kempf KK, et al. Treatment of a central arteriovenous malformation

of the mandible with cyanoacrylate: a 4-year follow-up. Oral Surg Oral Med Oral Pathol 1988; 65:267–71.

[24] Enjolras O, Mulliken JB, Boon LM, et al. A rare cutaneous anomaly. Plast Reconstr Surg 2001; 107:1647–54.

[25] Wisnicki JL. Hemangiomas and vascular malformations. Ann Plast Surg 1984;12:41–59.

[26] Enjolras O, Mulliken JB. Clinical and laboratory investigations: the current management of vascular birthmarks. Pediatr Dermatol 1993;10(4): 311–33.

[27] Eerola I, Boon LM, Watanabe S, et al. Locus for susceptibility for familial capillary malformation ("port-wine stain") maps to 5q. Eur J Hum Genet 2002;10:375–80.

[28] Breugem CC, Alders M, Salieb-Beugelaar GB, et al. A locus for hereditary capillary malformations mapped on chromosome 5q. Hum Genet 2002;110:343–7.

[29] Eerola I, Boon LM, Mulliken JB, et al. Capillary malformation-arteriovenous malformation, a new clinical and genetic disorder caused by RASA1 mutations. Am J Hum Genet 2003;73:1240–9.

[30] Vikkula M, Boon LM, Carraway KL 3rd, et al. Vascular dysmorphogenesis caused by an activating mutation in the receptor tyrosine kinase TIE2. Cell 1996;87:1181–90.

[31] Gallione CJ, Pasyk KA, Boon LM, et al. A gene for familial venous malformations maps to chromosome 9p in a second large kindred. J Med Genet 1995;32:197–9.

[32] Calvert JT, Riney TJ, Kontos CD, et al. Allelic and locus heterogeneity in inherited venous malformations. Hum Mol Genet 1999;8:1279–89.

[33] Mulliken JB. Vascular birthmarks: hemangiomas and malformations. Philadelphia: Saunders; 1988. p. 301–42.

[34] Burrows PE, Fellows KE. Techniques for management of pediatric vascular anomalies. In: Cope C, editor. Current techniques in interventional radiology. Philadelphia: Current Medicine; 1995. p. 12–27.

[35] Dubois JM, Sebag GH, De Prost Y, et al. Soft-tissue venous malformations in children: percutaneous sclerotherapy with Ethibloc. Radiology 1991;180:195–8.

[36] Anavi Y, Har-El G, Mintz S. The treatment of facial haemangioma by percutaneous injections of sodium tetradecyl sulfate. J Laryngol Otol 1988; 102:87–90.

[37] De Lorimier AA. Sclerotherapy for venous malformations. J Pediatr Surg 1995;30:188–93.

[38] Goebel WM, Lucatorto FM. Sodium tetradecyl sulfate treatment of benign vascular anomalies. J Oral Med 1976;31:76–80.

[39] Yakes WF, Haas DK, Parker SH, et al. Symptomatic vascular malformations: ethanol embolotherapy. Radiology 1989;170:1059–66.

[40] Gelbert F, Enjolras O, Deffrenne D, et al. Percutaneous sclerotherapy for venous malformation of the lips: a retrospective study of 23 patients. Neuroradiology 2000;42(9):692–6.

[41] Waner M, Suen J. Hemangiomas and vascular malformations of the head and neck. New York: Wiley-Liss; 1999.

[42] Van der Putte SC. The development of the lymphatic system in man. Adv Anat Embryol Cell Biol 1975;51:3–60.

[43] Gorenstein A, Katz S, Rein A, et al. Giant cystic hygroma associated with venous aneurysm. J Pediatr Surg 1992;27:1504–6.

[44] Joseph AE, Donaldson JS, Reynolds M. Neck and thorax venous aneurysm: association with cystic hygroma. Radiology 1989;170:109–12.

[45] Ogita S, Tsuto T, Deguchi E, et al. OK-432 therapy for unresectable lymphangiomas in children. J Pediatr Surg 1991;26:263–70.

[46] Giguere CM, Bauman NM, Sato Y, et al. Treatment of lymphangiomas with OK-432 (Picibanil) sclerotherapy: a prospective multi-institutional trial. Arch Otolaryngol Head Neck Surg 2002;128(10):1137–44.

[47] Rautio R, Keski-Nisula L, Laranne J, et al. Treatment of lymphangiomas with OK-432 (Picibanil). Cardiovasc Intervent Radiol 2003;26(1):31–6.

NEUROIMAGING
CLINICS
OF NORTH AMERICA

Neuroimag Clin N Am 17 (2007) 239–244

ELSEVIER
SAUNDERS

Cerebral Sinovenous Thrombosis in Children

Tali Jonas Kimchi, MD[a], Seon Kyu Lee, MD, PhD[a],*, Ronit Agid, MD[a],
Manohar Shroff, MD[b], Karel G. Ter Brugge, MD[a]

- Epidemiology
- Pathophysiology
- Risk factors
- Imaging

- Symptoms
- Treatment
- Outcome
- References

Cerebral venous thrombosis usually involves the cerebral venous sinuses, such as superior sagittal sinus and transverse sinus, but may involve deep venous system or cerebral cortical veins with isolated form or as part of a diffuse thrombotic process. Sinovenous thrombosis (SVT) in children is rare, and the symptoms and signs are nonspecific especially in the neonatal population. Thus, the diagnosis of SVT could be delayed or easily misdiagnosed. However, recent growing clinical awareness and improved noninvasive imaging techniques such as MR imaging have allowed us to diagnose the SVT in children earlier and more promptly.

Epidemiology

It is estimated that SVT constitutes approximately 20% of ischemic cerebral vascular disease in children. The incidence of SVT was 0.67 cases per 100,000 children per year between term birth to 18 years old. In that group, 43% of children who had SVT were neonates, and 54% were less then 1 year old, showing 97% of children who had SVT

were developed within a year after birth [1]. Carvalho and colleagues [2] described a group of 31 children who had SVT; the median age of this group was 14 days, and 61% of patients were neonates. The incidence of the SVT is likely to increase with certain medical conditions, including prematurity, leukemia, and heart disease. Improvements in neuroimaging techniques such as MR venography and CT venography also contribute to a rise in the incidence of SVT [3].

Pathophysiology

Thrombosis of the venous system can occur due to venous stasis, prothrombotic status, involvement of the vessel wall, and endovascular deposition of embolic materials. A slow blood flow also favors the formation and propagation of thrombus in the venous system.

Venous infarction can occur when the pressure in the venous system rises above the arterial perfusion pressure. Thus, possible mechanism of venous infarction in SVT could be explained as follows. The

[a] Division of Neuroradiology, Toronto Western Hospital, Department of Medical Imaging, University Health Network (UHN), University of Toronto, Toronto, Ontario, Canada
[b] Division of Neuroradiology, Department of Radiology, Hospital for Sick Children, University of Toronto, 555 University Avenue, Toronto, Ontario, Canada M5G 1X8
* Corresponding author. Department of Medical Imaging, Toronto Western Hospital, Suite 3MC-429, #399 Bathurst Street, Toronto, ON, M5T2S8, Canada.
E-mail address: seonkyu.lee@uhn.on.ca (S.K. Lee).

1052-5149/07/$ – see front matter © 2007 Elsevier Inc. All rights reserved.
neuroimaging.theclinics.com

doi:10.1016/j.nic.2007.01.006

obstruction of venous outflow due to the venous thrombosis raises the venous pressure in the area of the brain that needs to be drained through the occluded vein or sinus (venous congestion). The local venous congestion leads to extravasations of fluid and blood into the brain parenchyma (hemorrhagic infarction). Hydrocephalus can be developed in the cases of major sinus thrombosis and occlusion probably due to impairment in the absorption of cerebrospinal fluid through the arachnoid granulations [4].

Risk factors

SVT may be associated with various local or systemic conditions, such as prematurity, leukemia, and heart disease. Children who have SVT frequently have risk factors that tend to be related to the patient's age. For example, only less than 5% of children who had SVT showed no predisposing risk factor [1].

Neonates are especially susceptible to SVT. Acute systemic illnesses were present in 84% of neonates in the Canadian stroke registry. The most frequently associated medical conditions include pre- or perinatal complications, such as asphyxia at birth, prolonged rupture of membranes, gestational diabetes, and maternal infections. Other neonatal conditions associated with SVT are dehydration, bacterial sepsis, meningitis, and various prothrombotic disorders. Although prothrombotic disorders were described in 15% to 20% of SVT in neonates [1,5,6], the contribution of those conditions to SVT is not clear. Fitzgerald and colleagues [7] demonstrated gestational/delivery factors were present in 82%, and other comorbid conditions, such as dehydration, sepsis, and cardiac defects, were present in 62% in a group of 42 children who had neonatal SVT.

In infants who have SVT, head and neck disorders were more common. Most head and neck disorders were infections related to otitis media and mastoiditis [1]. Iron-deficiency anemia is frequently associated with SVT in older children. Sébire and colleagues [8] reported that 62% of children who had SVT, aged 3 weeks to 13 years, had anemia and/or microcytosis including iron deficiency, hemolytic, sickle cell, and β-thalassaemia. In older children who have SVT, chronic systemic diseases are present in approximately 40% to 60% of cases. These include cardiac diseases, connective tissue disorders, inflammatory bowel diseases, hematologic disorders, and nephrotic syndrome [8,9]. Children who have chronic illnesses are prone to develop sinovenous thrombosis, probably secondary to an acquired hypercoagulable state. Acute illnesses like sepsis or dehydration are also important in the older age group of children. Recent head trauma and recent surgery that resulted in sinus damage represent approximately 13% of SVT cases [8].

Prothrombotic disorders, whether acquired or inherited, are important in the pathogenesis of SVT in children. Patients who have a malignant tumor such as non-Hodgkin lymphoma, leukemia, and neuroblastoma, may have various coagulation abnormalities leading to a prothrombotic state. Chemotherapy may also be associated with SVT.

Tests for prothrombotic disorders have revealed abnormalities in approximately 30% to 65% of children, including the presence of anticardiolipin antibodies; lupus anticoagulant; factor V Leiden; or the prothrombine-gene mutations; and decreased level of Protein C, antithrombin, Protein S, fibrinogen, or plasminogen [1,6,8,10]. Among them, anticardiolipin antibody is the most frequently acquired abnormality, and the presence of factor V Leiden is the most frequent genetic abnormality [1]. The acquired prothrombotic states seem to be more frequent then the inherited. The acquired deficiencies can include decreased level of antithrombin, protein C, protein S, anticardiolipin antibody, or lupus anticoagulant. They may be caused by an acquired disorder, such as infection, liver disease, nephrotic syndrome, or disseminated intravascular coagulation [1,11]. The impact of congenital prothrombotic disorders such as factor V Leiden mutation or prothrombin mutation 20210 in children who have SVT is less clear [8,10]. At all ages, there is a combination of a prothrombotic disorder and an acute illness in patients who have SVT.

Malformations of the sinuses and intracranial arteriovenous shunts, such as vein of Galen aneurysmal malformation (VGAM) or dural arteriovenous shunts are also known to induce or be associated with SVT.

Arteriovenous shunts and malformations of the dural sinuses may be seen before or at the time of the thrombotic episode. These vascular disorders can be combined with a coagulation disorder. A recent patient who had VGAM in our series who was completely treated by endovascular technique developed venous thrombosis episode. This episode is "unrelated" to the previously treated arteriovenous shunt, but a factor V Leiden deficit was confirmed after subsequent investigations. Another child presented with focal seizures related to parietal lobe cortical venous thrombosis few years after complete exclusion of his VGAM. Thus, venous thrombosis could be a responsible mechanism for various clinical episodes in the natural history of VGAM, cerebral arteriovenous malformation, dural arteriovenous shunt, dural sinus malformation, and even maxillofacial arteriovenous malformation.

Imaging

Widespread availability of power doppler ultrasound, contrast enhanced CT, and MR imaging, has resulted in increased and earlier diagnosis of SVT in children. The conventional angiography is rarely performed to make such diagnosis. The degree of clinical suspicion, the quality of the examination, and the radiologic interpretation can impact the accuracy of these imaging studies.

MR imaging and MR venogaphy (Fig. 1) seems to be the most sensitive for accurate diagnosis of dural sinus thrombosis; however, it could be nearly equal for other modalities such as CT and CT venography (Fig. 2) as well as ultrasound examinations in centers of imaging excellence. Detection of cortical vein thrombosis without dural sinus thrombosis either requires detailed MR imaging examination with special sequences or careful selective cerebral angiography. Conventional cerebral angiography can document the extension of the lesion and the quality of the venous collateral pathways. Because of their noninvasive nature, the MR and CT venography can be used as excellent follow-up imaging modalities.

In the cohort of 160 pediatric patients who had SVT, the location of the thrombosis was superficial in 86% and deep in 38% with no significant differences between neonates and nonneonates [1]. Multiple sinuses were involved in 49%, whereas the lateral sinus was more frequently involved in nonneonates (60%) than in neonates (39%). Cerebral parenchymal infarcts were present in 41%, which were hemorrhagic in more then 75%. Extraparenchymal hemorrhage was documented in 9%.

Symptoms

The presenting clinical features of SVT in children are age dependent and can vary from minimal and nonspecific symptoms such as decreased oral intake and irritability to more ominous signs such as lethargy and coma. Seizures, fever, lethargy, or irritability and respiratory distress are common signs

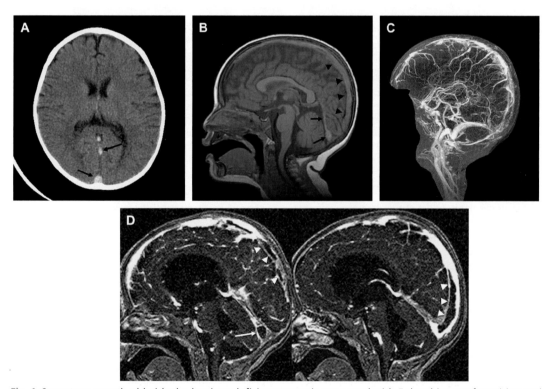

Fig. 1. Seventeen-month-old girl who has iron deficiency anemia presented with 5 days history of vomiting and dehydration and decreased consciousness level. (A) Noncontrast enhanced brain CT scan shows high attenuation of torcular helophili and straight sinus (*arrows*) without any brain parenchcymal abnormality. (B) Sagittal T1–weighted image shows increased signal intensity of superior sagittal sinus (*arrowheads*) as well as straight sinus (*arrows*), suggesting subacute hematoma. (C) Reconstructed Gd-enhanced MR venography using maximum intensity projection technique demonstrates nonvisualilzation of straight sinus and distal superior sagittal sinus. (D) Two consecutive source images of MR venography show multifocal filling defects in distal superior sagittal sinus (*white arrowheads*) and torcular (*white arrow*) indicating thrombus.

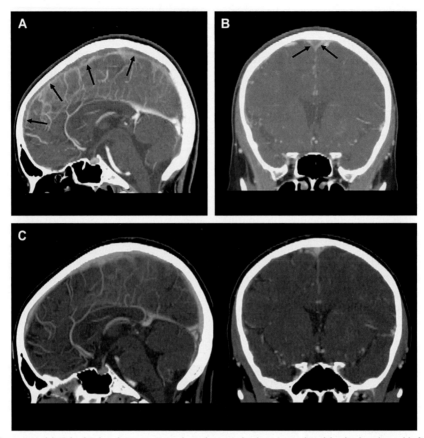

Fig. 2. Twelve-year-old girl who has known acute lymphocytic leukemia and suddenly developed left-side numbness, weakness, and dysarthria after having L-asparaginase as part of induction chemotherapy. (*A*) Sagittal reconstruction image of CT venography shows nonenhancing lesion replaces almost entire length of superior sagittal sinus (*arrows*). (*B*) Coronal reconstruction demonstrated triangular-shaped filling defects at superior sagittal sinus "empty delta sign" (*arrows*). (*C*) Follow-up CT venography after 3 months of low molecular weight heparin treatment demonstrated complete resolution of superior sagittal sinus thrombus.

of SVT in neonates. Older children commonly present with fever and lethargy, often associated with the classic signs of intracranial hypertension such as vomiting, headaches, papiledema, and abducens palsy [2]. In the Canadian pediatric cohort of SVT, 58% of children had seizures, 76% had diffuse neurologic signs, and 42% had focal neurologic deficits [1]. The symptomatology or natural history seems to be closely related to the patient's age.

If the SVT develops slowly, the patient may only have signs of chronic outflow obstruction, such as macrocrania, bruit, or enlarged facial veins [12]. Progressive lateral or sigmoid sinus thrombosis may result in benign intracranial hypertension, macrocrania with facial collateral venous circulation, or optic atrophy.

The initial symptoms of pseudotumor cerebri syndrome in older children and adolescents are typically headaches, sometimes accompanied by nausea and vomiting. However, young children may present with irritability rather than headaches. Some children are asymptomatic; their papilledema may be discovered at a routine school eye examination. Pseudotumor cerebri can also be manifest in infants as somnolence or apathy. Ataxia and dizziness are early symptoms in some childhood cases. The ataxia is intermittent. Neck, shoulder, or back pain may occur. Seizures and possibly ictal twitching of one hand have been reported. Paresthesias, facial numbness, tinnitus, and limb numbness have also been described.

The onset of the process—its acute extension versus its slowly progressive development, which enabled the collateral venous system to develop—may give rise to different syndromes. In some instances, although the dural sinuses are patent, the cerebral venous pattern at angiography suggests thrombosis of the cerebral veins. In Sturge-Weber disease, occlusion of the cortical vein is well recognized and is an important part of the disorder. It is often impossible to assess whether the cerebral vein thrombosis is isolated or secondary to a spontaneously recanalized sinus thrombosis or transdural vein thrombosis. The authors have seen sinuses spontaneously reopened in infants who have VGAM.

Craniostenosis, like other skull-base diseases, can produce occlusion of the basal sinuses and therefore produce a SVT syndrome. However, when bilateral, it rapidly leads to hydrodynamic disorders rather than venous ischemic syndrome to the brain. Transcranial outlets are recruited to bypass the obstacles of venous drainages. In these circumstances, the scalp and facial veins are draining the normal brain; thus these veins should be preserved during surgery.

Treatment

General medical and neurologic supportive care is the mainstay of treatment. Adequate hydration is critical, and aggressive antiepileptic and antibiotic therapy should be used when appropriate.

The usual treatment of acute SVT in adults involves early intervention in the process by means of anticoagulation therapy [13–15]. However, there are limited data regarding the efficacy and safety of systemic anticoagulation and fibrinolysis in pediatric SVT. A pilot study involving 30 children who had SVT, with a median age of 6 years, demonstrated that anticoagulant therapy, in particular lower molecular weight heparin, was safe and may have a role in the management of children who have SVT [5].

In a Canadian cohort of pediatric patients who had SVT, 53% received antithrombotic therapy, which represented 36% of the neonates and 66% of the nonneonates. Most children were treated for a 3-month period, and none of these died or had neurologic deterioration due to hemorrhagic complications. Seventy four percent of the neonates required anticonvulsant therapy as compared with 42% of the nonneonates who had SVT [1]. The role of surgery is by at large limited to mastoidectomy and shunt placement.

The role for fibrinolytic therapy by retrograde transvenous approach performed in adults who are not responding to anticoagulant therapy [16–18] is still rarely performed in the pediatric population with SVT.

Outcome

The outcome of pediatric patients who have acute SVT is highly variable, and reports in the literature are often of limited value because of the small number of patients receiving adequate follow-up assessments [2].

A cohort of 143 children in which neurologic outcome after SVT could be assessed with a mean follow-up of 1.6 years, included 61 neonates and 82 nonneonates. Fifty four percent were neurologically normal at follow-up; 38% had neurologic deficits; and 8% died, with half of the deaths being directly related to SVT [1]. Predictors for adverse neurologic outcome include seizures at presentation for nonneonates and the presence of infarcts in neonates and nonneonates. Thirteen percent of children had symptomatic recurrent thrombosis.

The long-term neurologic of sinovenous thrombosis in children is still unclear. However, the best available estimate suggests that after a mean of 2 years, approximately 75% of neonates and 50% of nonneonates will be neurologically normal [19–21].

It is not currently possible to predict which patients will recover with the best medical therapy. In addition, it seems to be reasonable to suppose that the poorer the patient's initial condition, the worse the prognosis will be. Thus, a more active medical treatment such as anticoagulation, which can take a certain degree of treatment-related risk, could be justified. It also seems reasonable to use an aggressive form of treatment such as retrograde transvenous fibrinolytic therapy in children whose condition declines despite adequate anticoagulation therapy.

References

[1] deVeber G, Andrew M, Adams C, et al. Cerebral sinovenous thrombosis in children. N Engl J Med 2001;345:417–23.

[2] Carvalho KS, Bodensteiner JB, Connolly PJ, et al. Cerebral venous thrombosis in children. J Child Neurol 2001;16:574–80.

[3] Casey SO, Alberico RA, Patel M, et al. Cerebral CT venography. Radiology 1996;198:163–70.

[4] Shroff M, deVeber G. Sinovenous thrombosis in children. Neuroimaging Clin N Am 2003;13: 115–38.

[5] deVeber G, Monagle P, Chan A, et al. Prothrombotic disorders in infants and children with cerebral thromboembolism. Arch Neurol 1998;55: 1539–43.

[6] Bonduel M, Sciuccati G, Hepner M, et al. Prethrombotic disorders in children with arterial ischemic stroke and sinovenous thrombosis. Arch Neurol 1999;56:967–71.

[7] Fitzgerald KC, Williams LS, Garg BP, et al. Cerebral sinovenous thrombosis in the neonate. Arch Neurol 2006;63(3):405–9.

[8] Sébire G, Tabarki B, Saunders DE, et al. Cerebral venous sinus thrombosis in children: risk factors, presentation, diagnosis and outcome. Brain 2005;128:477–89.

[9] Fluss J, Geary D, deVeber G. Cerebral sinovenous thrombosis and idiopathic nephrotic syndrome in childhood: report of four new cases and review of the literature. Eur J Pediatr 2006;165(10):709–16.

[10] Heller C, Heinecke A, Junker R, et al. Cerebral venous thrombosis in children. A multifactorial origin. Circulation 2003;108:1362–7.

[11] Ganesan V, Kelsey H, Cookson J, et al. Activated protein C resistance in childhood stroke. Lancet 1996;96:260.

[12] Pruvost P, Lasjaunias P, Rodesch G, et al. Benign pulsatile cranial bruit in children. Apropos of 6 cases. Arch Fr Pediatr 1989;46(8):579–82 [in French].

[13] Bousser MG. Cerebral venous thrombosis: diagnosis and management. J Neurol 2000;247:252–8.

[14] Einhaupl KM, Villringer A, Meister W, et al. Heparin treatment in sinus venous thrombosis. Lancet 1991;338:597–600.

[15] de Bruijn SF, Stam J. Randomized, placebo-controlled trial of anticoagulant treatment with low-molecular-weight heparin for cerebral sinus thrombosis. Stroke 1999;30:484–8.

[16] Tsai FY, Higashida RT, Matovich V, et al. Acute thrombosis of the intracranial dural sinus: direct thrombolytic treatment. AJNR Am J Neuroradiol 1992;13:1137–41.

[17] Horowitz M, Purdy P, Unwin H, et al. Treatment of dural sinus thrombosis using selective catheterization and urokinase. Ann Neurol 1995;38:58–67.

[18] Lee SK, Kim BS, Terbrugge K. Clinical presentation, imaging and treatment of cerebral venous thrombosis (CVT). Interventional Neuroradiology 2002;8:5–14.

[19] deVeber GA, MacGregor D, Curtis R, et al. Neurological outcome in survivors of childhood arterial ischemic stroke and sinovenous thrombosis. J Child Neurol 2000;15:316–24.

[20] Shevell MI, Silver K, O'Gorman AM, et al. Neonatal dural sinus thrombosis. Pediatr Neurol 1989;5:161–5.

[21] Barron TF, Gusnard DA, Zimmerman RA, et al. Cerebral venous thrombosis in neonates and children. Pediatr Neurol 1992;8:112–6.

NEUROIMAGING
CLINICS
OF NORTH AMERICA

Neuroimag Clin N Am 17 (2007) 245–258

Segmental Neurovascular Syndromes in Children

T. Krings, MD, PhD[a,b,*], S. Geibprasert, MD[a,c], C.B. Luo, MD[d],
J.J. Bhattacharya, MD[e], H. Alvarez, MD[a], Pierre Lasjaunias, MD, PhD[a]

In 1879, Sturge [1] reported a case that had an extensive port wine stain of the right face and head with a right-sided buphthalmus and a seizure attack. He also found a vascular malformation involving the ipsilateral brain. The atrophy of the affected cerebral hemisphere was suggested first by Weber [2] in 1922 by using radiograph examinations of the skull. In 1936, Bergstrand and colleagues [3] coined the currently accepted eponym Sturge-Weber disease and illustrated its pathologic characteristics, clinical manifestations, and surgical indications. Similarly,

an association between arteriovenous malformations (AVMs) of the face, retina, and brain was recognized first by Bonnet, Dechaume, and Blanc [4], in Lyon, France, who reported two cases in 1937. Six years later, Wyburn-Mason [5] reviewed all similar cases previously described and, in a detailed study, added nine more examples. The association of retinal, facial, and cerebral vascular malformations became known as Bonnet-Dechaume-Blanc syndrome in France and continental Europe, and as Wyburn-Mason syndrome in the English

[a] Service de Neuroradiologie Diagnostique et Thérapeutique, Hôpital Bicêtre, 78, rue du Général Leclerc, 94275 Le Kremlin-Bicêtre, Paris, France
[b] Department of Neuroradiology, University Hospital, University of Technology, Aachen, Pauwelsstrasse 30, 52057 Aachen, Germany
[c] Department of Rradiology, Ramathibodi Hospital, Rama 6 Rd, 10400 Bangkok, Thailand
[d] Department of Radiology, Taipei Veterans General Hospital, 201 Shih-Pai Road, 112 Taipei, Taiwan
[e] Department of Neuroradiology, Institute of Neurological Sciences, Southern General Hospital, 1345 Govan Road, Glasgow, G51 4TF, UK
* Corresponding author. Department of Neuroradiology, University Hospital, University of Technology, Aachen, Pauwelsstrasse 30, 52057 Aachen, Germany.
E-mail address: tkrings@izkf.rwth-aachen.de (T. Krings).

doi:10.1016/j.nic.2007.02.006

literature. Because the degree of expression of the syndromes' components varies, both clinically and morphologically, some confusion existed regarding the use of the two names. The term Bonnet-Dechaume-Blanc was sometimes preferred for the more extreme end of the disease spectrum, which includes high-flow maxillofacial AVMs. However, careful reading of the original articles confirms that both descriptions were referring to the same condition; thus, both eponyms can be used interchangeably.

The association between AVMs of the spinal cord and the skin was named after Stanley Cobb, a resident under Harvey Cushing, who in 1915 described the case of an 8-year-old boy who presented with acute paraplegia and had a skin discoloration of the same metamere, identified as a nevus. On surgery, a large spinal AVM was noticed.

Lastly, the association of cervicofacial hemangiomas with vascular and nonvascular intracranial malformations was recognized first by Pascual-Castroviejo [6,7] who, in 1978, proposed the name "cutaneous hemangioma-vascular complex syndrome." In 1996, Frieden and colleagues [8] proposed the acronym PHACE for this neurocutaneous syndrome; this acronym is derived from the spectrum of clinical findings that can be displayed in affected patients, (ie, *P*osterior cranial fossa malformations, *H*emangiomas, *A*rterial anomalies, *C*oarctation of the aorta and cardiac defects, and abnormalities of the *E*ye).

All the previously mentioned syndromes have been classified as neurocutaneous syndromes or phakomatoses. Within the past few years, however, the classic view of these phakomatoses has been revisited, and they no longer can be discussed without taking into consideration the recent genetic or biologic contributions that have suggested the neural crest and disorders in cephalic migration as a common link between the various components of many of these syndromes.

In this article, the authors first describe the concept of cephalic migration and then, based on this concept (ie, using a metameric approach), try to elucidate the previously mentioned syndromes and their common link.

General concepts: neural crest, cephalic migration, and the arterial-veno-lymphatic tree

The neural crest and neural plate share a common lineage. Cells of the lateral border of the developing neural plate (ie, the neural folds), under the inductive influence of the adjacent epithelium and possibly the mesoderm, develop into crest cells; hence, their common metameric origin with the cells of the hindbrain [9,10]. Moreover, it appears that all neural plate cells can become crest cells given the appropriate signals, and vice versa, and even epithelial cells can, in vitro, contribute to the neural crest lineage. They also share a metameric relationship with the adjacent cephalic mesoderm. The neural crest gives rise to a wide range of cell types, including skin, connective tissue, the skeleton of the craniofacial region, forebrain meninges, and the tunica media of the blood vessels of the face and forebrain (the endothelial cells here and elsewhere are derived from mesoderm). In recent years, the Hox genes–controlled segmentation of the rhombencephalon into rhombomeres, and of the forebrain into prosomeres [11,12] has been substantiated in birds, mice, and other animals, and extrapolated to humans [13]. After Le Douarin's [14,15] introduction of the quail-chick chimera system in 1969, which allows labelling of cells in avian embryos and then following their migration to their definitive sites, studies have revealed the metameric nature of brain and craniofacial structures deriving mainly from the neural crest and plate [16]. The initial process of vessel formation in the embryo, known as vasculogenesis, involves differentiation and sprouting of mesoderm-derived endothelial cells to form the primitive capillary network, which is then extended and remodeled by angiogenesis [14]. These primary capillary vessels progressively become ensheathed by differentiating smooth muscle cells. Although head and neck endothelial cells, as elsewhere, derive from mesoderm, the tunica media of these vessels differentiates from neural crest cells [17], which stream into the developing head and pharyngeal arches. Hox gene–encoded positional information in the crest cells is known to be involved in patterning of the pharyngeal arches, and is most likely involved also in determining the neural crest cell distribution among the arch-derived arteries. The work of Couly and colleagues [18] has shown further that the neural crest and mesodermal cells originating from a given transverse (metameric) level of the embryo finally occupy the same territory in the head, and that these embryonic tissues are regionalized in various areas devoted to providing blood vessels to specific regions of the face and brain.

A somatic mutation developing in the region of the neural crest or adjacent cephalic mesoderm before migration could, therefore, be expected to produce malformations with a segmental distribution. In fact, in avian experiments, fate maps of the cells occupying specific regions of the neural plate, crest, and cephalic mesoderm revealed striking similarities to the distribution of lesions encountered, for example, in the Wyburn-Mason syndrome (Fig. 1) [19].

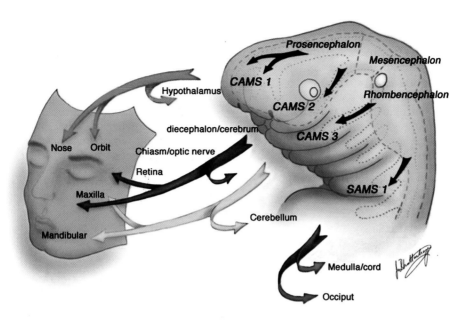

Fig. 1. Cerebrofacial vascular metameric syndromes. Three territories linking the brain to the face can be recognized. Depending on the type of cell involved, arteriovenous (CAMS 1–3) or venolymphatic (CVMS 1–3) metameric syndromes can be present. At the first cervical segment SAMS are represented. (SAMS 1; *green arrow*). The linkages between the different territories described in the figures are derived from fate maps of the cells occupying specific regions of the neural plate, crest, and cephalic mesoderm. (*From* Bhattacharya JJ, Luo CB, Suh DC, et al. Wyburn-Mason or Bonnet-Dechaume-Blanc as cerebrofacial arteriovenous metameric syndromes (CAMS) a new concept and a new classification. Interventional Neuroradiology 2001;7:5–17; with permission.)

In addition to their similarities in segmental distribution pattern and their link to the concept of neural crest development, metameric origins of cells, and cephalic migration, these segmental vascular syndromes share features such as their evolutive nature over time and their potential incomplete expression. The former may lead to a progressive enlargement of some of the lesions, revealing potential angiogenic activity, or to a progressive expression in time. The latter demonstrates that all features of a specific syndrome may not be found at clinical presentation, because of differences in vulnerability, the specificity of the triggering event, or incomplete expression, as described earlier. Despite these similarities, the main difference between the herewith described segmental vascular syndromes (namely, cerebrofacial venous metameric syndromes [CVMS] [20], cerebrofacial or spinal arteriovenous metameric syndromes [CAMS or SAMS] [19], and PHACE syndrome [PHACES] [21]) is the target of the lesion found on different regions of the arterio-venous tree: on the venolymphatic end in CVMS, on the capillary-venous side in CAMS and SAMS, and on the arterial-capillary end in PHACES. Although the timing of the triggering event to produce a metameric syndrome as described in this article is the same (fourth to fifth embryonic week), the target differs. Arteries and

veins are not identified by flow characteristics, but reveal their differences early by molecular properties. A specific trigger is therefore likely to be selective enough to differentiate between the more arterial and the more venous target, which is why, for example, port wine stains are not associated with intracranial AVMs. A striking difference between CVMS and CAMS on the one side and PHACES on the other is that, although all three syndromes share the migrating pattern of the neural crest and cephalic mesoderm along their three main paths, the clinical manifestations associated with PHACES (ie, disorders at the level of the sternum, the aorta, the internal carotid and intracranial arteries, the eye, and the posterior fossa) suggest a longitudinal dysfunction of the cephalic neural crest and are different from the axial, segmentally arranged vascular syndromes found in CAMS and CVMS, with lesions found within a single metamere (see Fig. 1). The association of hemangiomas in the cerebello-pontine angle with ipsilateral agenesis of the internal carotid, as described later, as potential manifestations of PHACES points to the link that exists in this syndrome between the third aortic arch, the third branchial arch, and the romboencephalic pattern of migration, also demonstrated in CAMS and CVMS. Finally, although CAMS and CVMS are well differentiated cranially (presumably because of their origin form the neural crest), sometimes they are not well delineated from each other at the spinal level (where the neural crest does not contribute directly to vasculogenesis). Therefore, the venolymphatic Klippel-Trenaunay syndrome may be associated with spinal cord arterial aneurysms (AA) and AVMs, whereas port wine stains (as a typical venous malformation) can be associated with typical SAMS (as a more arterial disease).

Cerebrofacial and spinal arteriovenous metameric syndromes

The association of AVMs of the brain, the orbit (retinal or retrobulbar lesions), and the maxillofacial region was named originally after Bonnet-Dechaume-Blanc and Wyburn-Mason. Because of the previously mentioned metameric concept of neural crest development, the authors have proposed a rational classification reflecting the putative underlying disorder, and have coined the acronym CAMS. Depending on the involved structures, several CAMS can be differentiated: CAMS 1 as a midline prosencephalic (olfactory) group with involvement of the hypothalamus, corpus callosum, hypophysis, and nose (Fig. 2); CAMS 2 as a lateral prosencephalic (optic) group with involvement of the optic nerve, retina, parieto-temporal-occipital lobes, thalamus, and maxilla (Fig. 3); and CAMS 3 as a rhombencephalic (otic) group with involvement of the cerebellum, pons, petrous bone, and mandible (Fig. 4). CAMS 3 is located in a strategic position on the crossroad between the complex cephalic segmental arrangements and the relatively simplified spinal metamers, and therefore it may bear transitional characteristics [22]. SAMS, previously referred to as Cobb's syndrome or spinal AVM of the juvenile type, likewise affects the whole myelomere; therefore, affected patients typically present with multiple shunts of the spinal cord,

nerve root, and bone, and paraspinal, subcutaneous, and skin tissues that share the same myelomere (Fig. 5) [23]. SAMS can be named from 1 to 31, depending on the affected myelomere [22]. A more extensive insult leads to overlapping territories, producing a complete prosencephalic phenotype (CAMS 1 + 2) or bilateral involvement. The insult producing the underlying lesion would have to develop before the migration occurs and, thus, before the fourth week of development. The disease spectrum may be incomplete either because some cells are spared or because they have not been triggered to reveal the disease [24], leading to cases without retinal involvement [25], cerebral involvement, or facial involvement [26]. Retinal AVM is often the earliest manifestation of a CAMS and in some cases follow-up has shown secondary expression of the full syndrome. In one case, the full extent of the spectrum was revealed over a 28-year period [27]. Anticipation of the other localizations can be discussed when isolated retinal, hypothalamic, or optic nerve AVM is diagnosed.

Retinal Arteriovenous Malformations and Arteriovenous Malformations Along the Optic Nerve and Chiasm

The most common presenting symptom of retinal AVMs and AVMs along the optic nerve and chiasm is visual deterioration (reduced acuity or field) because retinal AVMs are present in most CAMS patients. These symptoms occur before the age of 18 in more than 50% of cases. Usually, retinal AVMs or arteriovenous communications of the retina (AVCR) are considered to be stable retinal lesions, despite progression of the coexisting intracranial AVMs [28]. Loss of vision may occur because of intraretinal macular hemorrhage, central and peripheral retinal vein occlusion, or vitreous hemorrhage; a gradual reduction of vision may be caused by neovascular glaucoma in association with changes in

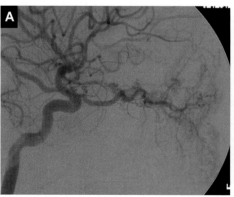
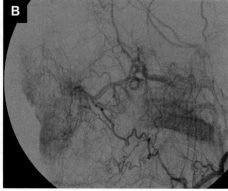

Fig. 2. CAMS1. Association of an olfactory AVM with a nasal AVM in a 12-year-old girl with recurrent severe epistaxis.

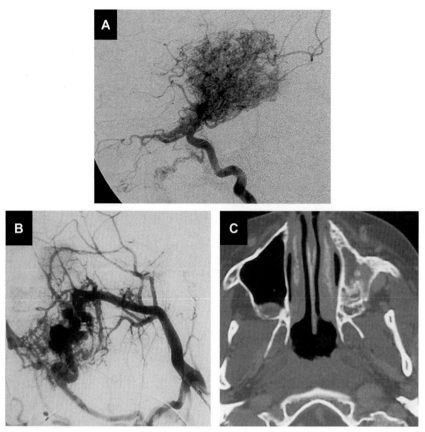

Fig. 3. CAMS 2. Associated thalamic hypothalamic left-sided AVM (*A*) in a 9-year-old girl with a decline in visual acuity of the left eye and an inferior quadrantanopia of the right visual field owing to a maxillofacial AVM (*B*) that led also to significant maxillar bone hypotrophy (*C*).

the retinal AVMs and retinal and choroidal ischemia [29]. The retinal AVM or AVCR is called a racemose hemangioma in the ophthalmologic literature (although racemose hemangioma is probably a misnomer because it does not exhibit proliferative behavior). Sometimes it is detected several years before further neurologic symptoms lead to more detailed investigations (CT, MR imaging) confirming the presence of a retinal AVM, but also revealing an associated brain AVM.

Optic nerve and chiasmatic AVMs are also hallmark findings in CAMS. They often appear to be clinically silent, eventually resulting in a slowly progressive, functional deficit. The presenting symptoms include decreased visual acuity and field defects, or blindness from optic nerve atrophy and progressive dysfunction of the optic pathways.

Exophthalmos is a rare presenting symptom in CAMS, with optic nerve AVMs and intraorbital congestion resulting in mass effect. Exophthalmos can also result from an enlarged ophthalmic vein, which may drain normal brain tissue, or from cerebral AVMs related to increased intracranial venous pressure caused by venous occlusion of draining intracranial veins.

Treatment (a combined surgical and endovascular approach) of these orbital lesions remains a challenge because of the complex anatomy and hemorrhagic characteristics of the malformation [30].

Cerebral Arteriovenous Malformations

Considered metameric lesions, intracranial AVMs in CAMS are one of the most common findings in such patients. Cerebral AVMs in CAMS may involve in continuity the corpus callosum, the olfactory region, and the hypothalamus (CAMS 1); the optic chiasm, the thalamus, and the cortex around the calcarine fissure (CAMS 2); or the cerebellum (CAMS 3). Infrequently, they present as multiple scattered lesions in the same segmental distribution. Considering the angioarchitecture of cerebral AVMs in CAMS, certain findings differ from "classic" AVMs: the AVM nidus in CAMS is a cluster of small vessels with intervening normal brain tissue, some degree of angiogenesis, and a small shunting

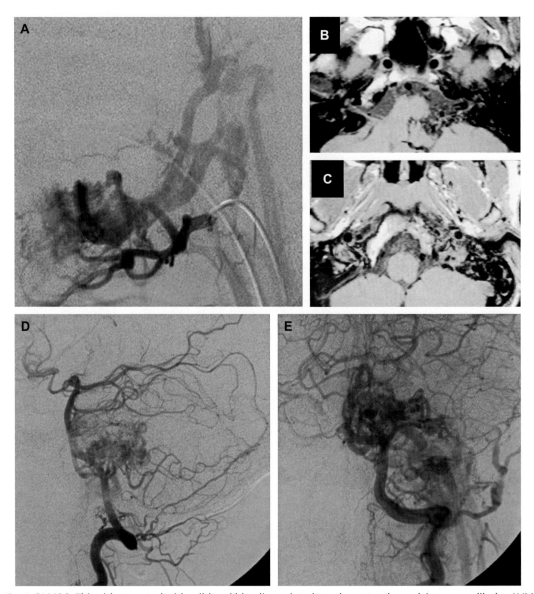

Fig. 4. CAMS 3. This girl presented with mild oral bleeding related to a loose tooth overlying a mandibular AVM (*A*). MR imaging (T1-weighted images precontrast) (*B, C*) reveals involvement of the brain of the ipsilateral posterior fossa, the subarachnoid space, and the temporal bone. Lateral view (*D*) and anteroposterior view (*E*) angiography of the vertebral artery demonstrate a cerebellar AVM.

volume [30]. Transdural arterial supply can be present. Progressive enlargement of these cerebral AVMs is one of the special observations in CAMS, suggesting that AVMs in CAMS are not static processes within the segment that carry the embryonic defect. Multifocality is another typical aspect of CAMS-associated AVMs. Despite the common occurrence of cerebral AVMs in CAMS, they are usually clinically silent or asymptomatic at the time of discovery. They rarely present with acute neurologic symptoms caused by intracerebral or subarachnoid hemorrhage [19]; rather, they reveal with progressive neurologic deterioration without evidence of intracranial bleeding, most likely owing to a progression in size. About 25% of patients who have CAMS-associated AVMs bleed during the course of their disease [30].

Therapeutic management of cerebral AVMs is particularly challenging. The authors suggest targeted embolization in an attempt to exclude weak angioarchitectural aspects or to reduce the arteriovenous (AV) shunt in the least eloquent areas in symptomatic patients who are significantly affected clinically. At present, brain AVMs are not considered curable because of their size, location, and natural history [30].

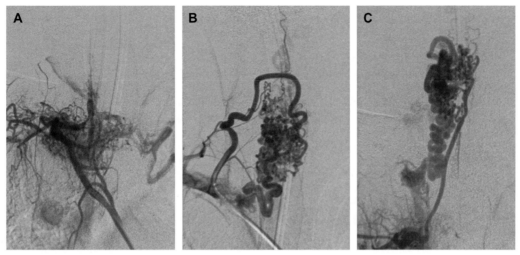

Fig. 5. SAMS. Typical aspect of SAMS 10 with T2 vertebral and soft tissue involvement, and corresponding myelomeric location of an intramedullary glomerular AVM fed by a radiculopial artery in a 9-year-old boy with progressive paraparesis.

Facial Arteriovenous Malformations, Nasal Arteriovenous Malformations, and Mandibular Arteriovenous Malformations

Nasal AVMs (CAMS 1), maxillofacial AVMs (CAMS 2), and mandibular AVMs (CAMS 3) are present in about one third of patients who have CAMS. The presence of the facial vascular lesion can be difficult to recognize or may be clinically silent, sometimes representing a small stable red spot or angioma since infancy or early childhood. Then, an unknown trigger occurs that promotes growth of the lesion, with revealing symptoms such as bleeding of the gums or mass effect, resulting in facial asymmetry, often during adolescence. Epistaxis may be encountered in high-flow maxillofacial AVMs. The angioarchitecture of facial or mandibular AVMs in CAMS looks similar to sporadic cases. Usually, they present as an arteriovenous fistula or nidustype AVM with intranidal fistulous compartments [30]. Large, proximal arterial aneurysms can be present, despite relative slow flow or small-sized facial or mandibular AVMs. Because sporadic, isolated maxillar or mandibular AVMs are not associated with external carotid artery (ECA) aneurysms regardless of their flow, facial AVMs in CAMS patients are different from their sporadic counterparts in terms of angioarchitecture and natural history. Maxillar or mandibular AVMs with intraosseous venous lakes or pouches are also at risk of gum bleeding and severe hemorrhages after tooth extraction [22,28,31]. The presence of atypical aneurysms on the ECA in CAMS patients points toward the angiogenic potential of this syndrome.

Cerebrofacial venous metameric syndromes

Encephalotrigeminal angiomatosis or Sturge-Weber syndrome (SWS) is a nonfamilial disease with a skin discoloration (port wine stain) in the V_1 territory, associated with a calcified leptomeningeal venous malformation of the ipsilateral supratentorial hemisphere [30]. Symptoms appear before the second year of age and include cosmetic and neurologic problems related to subjacent cerebral atrophy, leading to epilepsy, deficits, and mental retardation. Port wine stains that represent localized dermal venular malformations are classically present. They usually remain stable and do not bleed, except when they involve the oral cavity or the pharynx. Although most port wine stains are isolated vascular anomalies, they may be associated with an underlying vascular malformation or a more complex dysmorphogenesis [32]. This facial vascular malformation usually is unilateral, but it can involve the midline, and is reported to extend to the chest, trunk, and limbs in some cases. In exceptional cases it can be bilateral [33]. Often, it is associated with progressive thickening of the skin and subcutaneous layers, and facial capillaryvenous malformations with subjacent lymphatic malformation; in such cases, overgrowth of the underlying facial skeleton is demonstrated, which may result in facial asymmetry and dental malocclusion. About one third of the patients who have SWS have ocular or orbital abnormalities such as choroid venous malformation, congenital glaucoma with enlargement of the globe (buphthalmus), optic disc colobomas, and cataract.

Intracranial manifestations generally are not present in patients who have port wine stains confined to the lower and midface area.

In fact, associated intracranial vascular anomalies in SWS consist of cortical venous thrombosis with capillary venous proliferation and enlargement of the transmedullary collateral venous drainage, with or without choroid plexus hypertrophy. Typical CT or MR imaging findings include gyral enhancement and a pronounced enhancement of the ipsilateral choroid plexus (Fig. 6) [34]. Occlusion of venules at the gyral crowns produces cortical calcifications and brain atrophy that may result in seizures and mental retardation [20,35]. MR imaging performed early during the course of the disease demonstrates normal, or even accelerated, myelination in the centrum semiovale on the involved hemisphere.

As in the other syndromes reported here, the venous abnormalities that affect the central nervous system and the face involve segmentally related territories [18]. The authors presume that SWS is expressed differently in the face, compared with the brain, because of the phenotypic cell identity acquired during mesenchymatous migration (from neural crest and cephalic mesoderm). Differences in the vascular abluminal environment, the exposure to different postnatal triggers, and changing vulnerabilities at different moments, all may lead to different phenotypic expressions, despite a common underlying disease. Thus, the venous malformations observed in SWS can be regarded as CVMS [20,36]. In some patients, this metameric syndrome may involve two or three consecutive metamers and may be more or less complete in all tissues derived at a given level. As seen in CAMS, different groups can be encountered: the medial prosencephalic group (olfactory) with involvement of the forehead and nose (CVMS 1); the lateral prosencephalic group (optic), with involvement of the occipital lobe, eye, cheek, and maxilla (CVMS 2); and the rhombencephalon (otic) group with involvement of the cerebellum, lower face, and mandible (CVMS 3). According to this grouping, one can see that the port wine stain is not along the trigeminal nerve territory

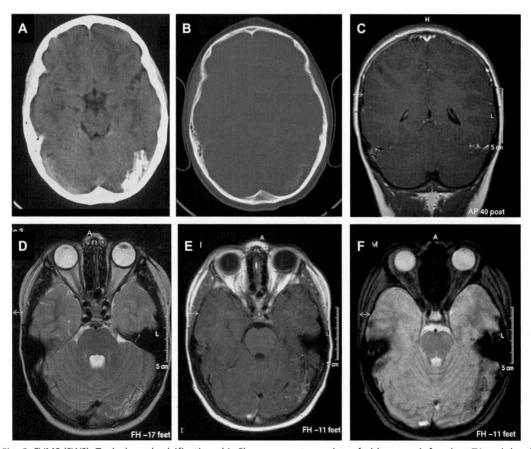

Fig. 6. CVMS (SWS). Typical gyral calcifications (*A, B*) are present as a sign of old venous infarction. T1-weighted images after contrast (*C, E*) demonstrate the gyral enhancement, whereas T2- (*D*) and T2*- (*F*) weighted images demonstrate pathologic vessels and calcifications.

distribution, but is, in fact, related to a mesoderm-neural crest region segmentation (Fig. 7). The classic form of SWS corresponds to CVMS 1 + 2, as a full prosencephalic impairment with the lesion affecting the orbit and maxillofacial region, whereas in the rare form of CVMS 3, the port wine stain is localized at the mandible with "bear-shaped" discoloration [20,36]. Being a segmental or metameric disorder, the full expression of CVMS includes port wine stains in one or several facial segments related to the migration of vascular cells from the mesoderm and neural crest, lymphangiomatous malformation of the cheek area, maxillofacial (malar, frontal, or maxilla) and skull base (ethmoid, sphenoid petrous) hypertrophy, and pial cortical venous occlusions (supra or infratentorial) with associated gyral calcifications and atrophy. An incomplete spectrum corresponding to the same cranial segmental disorder is encountered more frequently than the full expression of the disease.

PHACES

PHACES is a rare, congenital, syndromal pediatric disorder with less than 150 cases reported in the literature and a broad spectrum of clinical manifestations [8,21,37–45]. As mentioned previously, its characteristics are posterior fossa malformations, hemangiomas, arterial anomalies, coarctation of the aorta, cardiac defects, eye abnormalities, and sternum/abdominal raphe defects. Recently, arterial intracranial stenoses have been added as an additional feature of this syndrome that might lead to pediatric strokes and a moyamoya-like appearance

of the distal internal carotid artery (ICA) (Figs. 8 and 9) [21]. Although the hallmark of PHACES is the large "plaque-like" facial hemangioma, the spectrum of associated clinical and imaging findings may be complete or incomplete, and most patients display only one or two extracutaneous manifestations.

Although its pattern of inheritance has not been established yet, there is a striking female predominance, with a female/male ratio of 9:1 [21]. In 1996, PHACES was described by Frieden and colleagues as a complete syndrome, yet most instances, apart from the facial hemangioma, typically have only one or two extracutaneous manifestations [8,46].

Posterior Fossa Malformations

Posterior cranial fossa malformations are present in 32% to 74% of patients who have PHACES and are represented by Dandy-Walker malformations and cerebellar hemisphere hypoplasia (which typically is homolateral to the facial hemangioma) [7,43]. Of all Dandy-Walker malformations studied by Hirsch and colleagues [47], 10% were associated with cutaneous hemangiomas. These cases also showed a high female predominance (9:1), which was not observed in the isolated posterior fossa malformation group [47]. This posterior fossa cystic malformation points to the third to fourth week of development [47]. The association of intracranial hemangioma in the posterior fossa with PHACES [48] and with cortical dysplasia has also been reported [49].

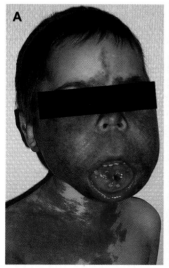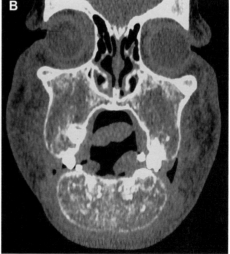

Fig. 7. CVMS (SWS). In this patient, a bilateral CVMS 2 and 3 is present, with maxillar and mandible involvement and hypertrophy.

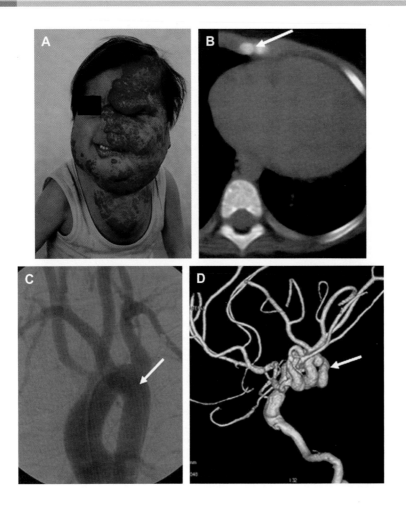

Fig. 8. PHACES. A 2-year-old child with an extensive left facial and upper thorax hemangioma (*A*). CT of the thorax (*B*) demonstrates the sternal cleft (*arrow*). The aortic arch angiography (*C*) reveals an aberrant course of the right subclavian artery (*arrow*). Three-dimensional digital subtraction angiography (DSA) (*D*) shows ectasia and elongation of the posterior division of the internal carotid artery (ICA) (*arrow*) and the C2 extracranial segment.

Hemangiomas

Hemangiomas are the most common benign tumors of infancy, occurring in up to 10% of children younger than 1 year of age [8]. Infantile hemangiomas are common vascular lesions that are usually solitary. Less than one half of the hemangiomas are present at birth; others appear in the first 3 months of life, with rapid growth until 6 to 8 months. A stable "plateau phase" is achieved between 8 and 12 months, followed by a slow involution that continues until 5 to 10 years of age [30]. Apart from this typical pattern, two variants can be encountered. One subgroup of hemangiomas appears as fully grown tumors shortly after birth and resolve rapidly, often leaving pronounced atrophic skin changes. This variant is known as "rapid involuting congenital (capillary) hemangioma" [50]. The second, albeit rare, variant is called "noninvoluting congenital (capillary) hemangioma"; it exhibits specific clinicopathologic and radiologic features and does not regress with time [51].

Facial hemangiomas can be classified as focal (tumor-like lesions) or diffuse (plaque-like lesions with segmental pattern). Diffuse lesions affect the mandibular segment in 38% of cases, the maxillary in 35% of cases, and the frontonasal in 27% of cases; however, in 24% of cases, more than one facial segment is involved [52]. Patients who have segmental distribution of lesions have a higher female/male ratio, almost twice that of patients who have focal lesions. In addition, segmental, plaque-like hemangiomas have been associated with PHACES [53].

Multiple hemangiomas of the skin (five or more) traditionally have been recognized as a clue to potential visceral hemangiomas, although this association also can be observed in segmental hemangiomas with less frequency [54]. Internal organ hemangiomas associated with multiple cutaneous hemangiomas is a known entity distinct from PHACES [37].

Hemangiomas in PHACES are typically plaque-like, ulcerated facial lesions that are not strictly segmented in distribution. One third of patients demonstrate cutaneous hemangiomas in regions apart from the head and neck.

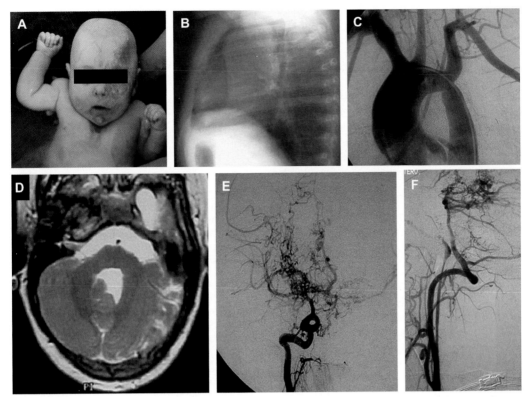

Fig. 9. PHACES. Left-sided facial hemangioma (*A*), aortic coarctation (*B*), posterior fossa malformation (*C*), sternal agenesis (*D*), narrowing of the ICA with a moyamoya-type revascularization (*E*) and arterial anomalies with segmental internal carotid artery (ICA) agenesis and type-1 proatlantal artery (*F*) are present in this child.

Cardiac Abnormalities and Aortic Coarctation

These anomalies are seen in approximately one third of cases, with coarctation being the most common abnormality. Typically encountered cardiac anomalies include right-sided aorta, persistent ductus arteriosus, ventriculo-septal defects, and pulmonary stenosis. It has been suggested that the side of the hemangioma and the side of the aortic arch abnormality, with or without coarctation, are associated (95% of concordance on ipsilaterality) [55].

Eye Abnormalities

Ophthalmologic findings are not as common as posterior fossa and arterial anomalies; however, colobomas, arcus corneae, optic nerve hypoplasia, increased retinal vascularity, and glaucoma have been described [56].

Sternal and Raphe Disorders

In addition to the various previously described structural cardiac abnormalities and aortic coarctation, ventral developmental defects such as sternal pits, sternal clefting, and supra-abdominal raphe should be looked for in suspected PHACES. Several investigators have speculated that the association of

sternal clefting and facial hemangiomas probably develops at between 8 and 10 weeks of gestational age. This association occurs in 7% of patients who have PHACES [8].

Arterial Anomalies

At least four different types of arterial anomalies seem to be associated with PHACES: agenesis of major cervical arteries, embryologic persistence of vessels, arterial stenoses, and the recently described dolicoectatic type of arterial segments [37].

The persistence of embryonic arteries, such as the trigeminal artery (often ipsilateral to the cutaneous hemangioma), occurs most commonly, followed by partial or complete agenesis of major cervical arteries, which usually also are ipsilateral to the cutaneous lesion. Other anomalies of the intracranial vasculature and the brain that have been described are hypoglossal, proatlantal, or stapedial persistence; segmental agenesis of the internal carotid artery with persistent basilar anastomosis; concomitant bilateral internal carotid artery agenesis; and vertebrobasilar system agenesis and cerebellopontine angle mass consistent with an intracranial hemangioma [30,48].

Segmental agenesis of the internal carotid artery is a common arterial abnormality found in PHACES [54]. Usually, flow is reconstituted in the adjacent distal internal carotid segment through embryonic vessels anastomoses, often involving the tympanic cavity.

Recently, stenoses have been described as a further feature of PHACES. In the series by Burrows and colleagues [46], the onset of occlusive disease was between birth and 18 months of age, which correlates with the proliferative phase of the hemangiomas, although in a previous study the subjects who had occlusive arterial disease were older (4 to 14 years of age) [21].

Recently, segmental arterial dolichoectasias have been found. These segmental dilatations are related to the segmental identity of the vessel with an associated segmental vulnerability, a condition inherent to a specific portion of the artery that is structurally more susceptible to suffering transformation when exposed to (or identified by) a trigger [37]. Topographic differences in the endothelial surface proteins and the vascular environment suggest a regional specificity of the vascular tree that may account for the specificity of the biologic response to a stimulus, although details of these biologic segmental differences remain poorly understood. During angiogenesis, various responses in a given (vulnerable) segment may be observed: increase in length (dolichoartery), centrifugal increase in diameter with lumen enlargement (aneurysm), or centripetal increase with lumen reduction (occlusion). The three types of response can coexist in contiguous segments, showing the difficulty in appreciating where the specificity of the trigger, the target edges, or the time intervenes to produce the detectable architectural change.

The authors therefore postulate that the different forms of arterial involvement in PHACES constitutes various phenotypes related to plurisegmental abnormal development of the neural crest involved in the dorsal aorta and cerebrofacial arterial structures. The timing of the revealing trigger might lead to different phenotypes, including agenesis (with concomitant embryologic persistence of vessels), stenoses, or elongation related to the same underlying vessel wall defect, and segmentally arranged proliferative activities mostly ipsilaterally distributed. The nature of the triggering event remains unclear, but because there is no evidence of a familial tendency, the authors presume a germline mutation unlikely.

The authors conclude that, although the diseases reported in this article may be rare, their relationships among each other, and their linkage with the development of the neural crest, may shed light on the complex and, as of yet, not fully understood pathology and etiology of various cerebral vascular disorders, and will, therefore, broaden knowledge about potential targets of treatment in the future.

References

[1] Sturge WA. A case of partial epilepsy apparently due to a lesion of one of the vasomotor centres of the brain. Transactions of the Clinical Society of London 1879;12:162–7.

[2] Weber FP. Right-sided hemihypertrophy resulting from right-sided congenital spastic hemiplegia. J Neurol Psychopathol 1922;3:134–9.

[3] Bergstrand H, Olivecrona H, Tonnis W. Gefässmissbildungen und Gefaessgeschwulste des Gehirns. Leipzig (Germany): Thieme; 1936.

[4] Bonnet P, Dechaume JP, Blanc E. L'anevrisme cirsoide de la retine. Ses relations avec l'anevrysme cirsoide du cerveau. Journal de Médecine de Lyon 1937;18:165–78 [in French].

[5] Wyburn-Mason R. Arteriovenous aneurysm of midbrain and retina, facial naevi and mental changes. Brain 1943;66:163–203.

[6] Pascual-Castroviejo I. Vascular and nonvascular intracranial malformation associated with external capillary hemangiomas. Neuroradiology 1978;16:82–4.

[7] Pascual-Castroviejo I, Viano J, Moreno F, et al. Hemangiomas of the head, neck, and chest with associated vascular and brain anomalies: a complex neurocutaneous syndrome. AJNR Am J Neuroradiol 1996;17:461–71.

[8] Frieden IJ, Reese V, Cohen D. PHACE syndrome. The association of posterior fossa brain malformations, hemangiomas, arterial anomalies, coarctation of the aorta and cardiac defects, and eye abnormalities. Arch Dermatol 1996;132:307–11.

[9] Baker CV, Bronner-Fraser M. The origins of the neural crest. Part I: embryonic induction. Mech Dev 1997;69:3–11.

[10] Baker CV, Bronner-Fraser M. The origins of the neural crest. Part II: an evolutionary perspective. Mech Dev 1997;69:13–29.

[11] Keynes R, Cook G, Davies J, et al. Segmentation and the development of the vertebrate nervous system. J Physiol (Paris) 1990;84:27–32.

[12] Lumsden A, Keynes R. Segmental patterns of neuronal development in the chick hindbrain. Nature 1989;337:424–8.

[13] Puelles L, Rubenstein JL. Expression patterns of homeobox and other putative regulatory genes in the embryonic mouse forebrain suggest a neuromeric organization. Trends Neurosci 1993;16:472–9.

[14] Le Douarin NM, Catala M, Batini C. Embryonic neural chimeras in the study of vertebrate brain and head development. Int Rev Cytol 1997;175:241–309.

[15] Le Douarin NM, Dieterlen-Lievre F, Teillet MA, et al. Interspecific chimeras in avian embryos. Methods Mol Biol 2000;135:373–86.

[16] Etchevers HC, Couly G, Vincent C, et al. Anterior cephalic neural crest is required for forebrain viability. Development 1999;126:3533–43.

[17] Risau W, Flamme I. Vasculogenesis. Annu Rev Cell Dev Biol 1995;11:73–91.

[18] Couly G, Coltey P, Eichmann A, et al. The angiogenic potentials of the cephalic mesoderm and the origin of brain and head blood vessels. Mech Dev 1995;53:97–112.

[19] Bhattacharya JJ, Luo CB, Suh DC, et al. Wyburn-Mason or Bonnet-Dechaume-Blanc as cerebrofacial arteriovenous metameric syndromes (CAMS) a new concept and a new classification. Interventional Neuroradiology 2001;7:5–17.

[20] Ramli N, Sachet M, Bao C, et al. Cerebrofacial venous metameric syndrome (CVMS) 3: Sturge-Weber syndrome with bilateral lymphatic/venous malformations of the mandible. Neuroradiology 2003;45:687–90.

[21] Bhattacharya JJ, Luo CB, Alvarez H, et al. PHACES syndrome: a review of eight previously unreported cases with late arterial occlusions. Neuroradiology 2004;46:227–33.

[22] Wong IY, Batista LL, Alvarez H, et al. Craniofacial arteriovenous metameric syndrome (CAMS) 3–a transitional pattern between CAM 1 and 2 and spinal arteriovenous metameric syndromes. Neuroradiology 2003;45:611–5.

[23] Krings T, Mull M, Gilsbach JM, et al. Spinal vascular malformations. Eur Radiol 2005;15:267–78.

[24] Bergwerff M, Verberne ME, DeRuiter MC, et al. Neural crest cell contribution to the developing circulatory system: implications for vascular morphology? Circ Res 1998;82:221–31.

[25] Brown DG, Hilal SK, Tenner MS. Wyburn-Mason syndrome. Report of two cases without retinal involvement. Arch Neurol 1973;28:67–9.

[26] Theron J, Newton TH, Hoyt WF. Unilateral retinocephalic vascular malformations. Neuroradiology 1974;7:185–96.

[27] Jiarakongmun P, Alvarez H, Rodesch G, et al. Clinical course and angioarchitecture of cerebrofacial arteriovenous metameric syndrome. Interventional Neuroradiology 2002;3:251–64.

[28] Yasuhara T, Ikeda T, Koizumi K, et al. Multiple cranial arteriovenous malformations in a child with eventual blindness in the affected eye. Am J Ophthalmol 1999;127:99–101.

[29] Effron L, Zakov ZN, Tomsak RL. Neovascular glaucoma as a complication of the Wyburn-Mason syndrome. J Clin Neuroophthalmol 1985;5:95–8.

[30] Lasjaunias P, Ter Brugge K, Berenstein A. Surgical neuroangiography. Berlin: Springer; 2006.

[31] Haw C, Sarma D, Ter Brugge K. Co-existence of mandibular arteriovenous malformation and cerebellar arteriovenous malformations. An example of cerebrofacial arteriovenous metameric syndrome type III. Interventional Neuroradiology 2003;9:71–4.

[32] Lin DD, Barker PB. Neuroimaging of phakomatoses. Semin Pediatr Neurol 2006;13:48–62.

[33] Baselga E. Sturge-Weber syndrome. Semin Cutan Med Surg 2004;23:87–98.

[34] Truhan AP, Filipek PA. Magnetic resonance imaging. Its role in the neuroradiologic evaluation of neurofibromatosis, tuberous sclerosis, and Sturge-Weber syndrome. Arch Dermatol 1993;129:219–26.

[35] Portilla P, Husson B, Lasjaunias P, et al. Sturge-Weber disease with repercussion on the prenatal development of the cerebral hemisphere. AJNR Am J Neuroradiol 2002;23:490–2.

[36] Luo C, Bhattacharya J, Ferreira M, et al. Cerebrofacial vascular disease. Orbit 2003;22:89–102.

[37] Baccin CE, Krings T, Alvarez H, et al. A report of two cases with dolichosegmental intracranial arteries as a new feature of PHACES syndrome. Childs Nerv Syst 2006, Epub ahead of print.

[38] Carles D, Pelluard F, Alberti EM, et al. Fetal presentation of PHACES syndrome. Am J Med Genet A 2005;132:110.

[39] Ceisler E, Blei F. Ophthalmic issues in hemangiomas of infancy. Lymphat Res Biol 2003;1:321–30.

[40] Goddard DS, Liang MG, Chamlin SL, et al. Hypopituitarism in PHACES association. Pediatr Dermatol 2006;23:476–80.

[41] Mazereeuw-Hautier J, Syed S, Harper JI. Sternal malformation/vascular dysplasia syndrome with linear hypopigmentation. Br J Dermatol 2006;155:192–4.

[42] Mazzie JP, Lepore J, Price AP, et al. Superior sternal cleft associated with PHACES syndrome: postnatal sonographic findings. J Ultrasound Med 2003;22:315–9.

[43] Rossi A, Bava GL, Biancheri R, et al. Posterior fossa and arterial abnormalities in patients with facial capillary haemangioma: presumed incomplete phenotypic expression of PHACES syndrome. Neuroradiology 2001;43:934–40.

[44] Ruiz-de-Luzuriaga AM, Bardo D, Stein SL. PHACES association. J Am Acad Dermatol 2006;55:1072–4.

[45] Vermeer S, van Oostrom CG, Boetes C, et al. A unique case of PHACES syndrome confirming the assumption that PHACES syndrome and the sternal malformation-vascular dysplasia association are part of the same spectrum of malformations. Clin Dysmorphol 2005;14:203–6.

[46] Burrows PE, Robertson RL, Mulliken JB, et al. Cerebral vasculopathy and neurologic sequelae in infants with cervicofacial hemangioma: report of eight patients. Radiology 1998;207:601–7.

[47] Hirsch JF, Pierre-Kahn A, Renier D, et al. The Dandy-Walker malformation. A review of 40 cases. J Neurosurg 1984;61:515–22.

[48] Judd CD, Chapman PR, Koch B, et al. Intracranial infantile hemangiomas associated with PHACE syndrome. AJNR Am J Neuroradiol 2007;28:25–9.

[49] Grosso S, De Cosmo L, Bonifazi E, et al. Facial hemangioma and malformation of the cortical development: a broadening of the PHACE

spectrum or a new entity? Am J Med Genet A 2004;124:192–5.

[50] Boon LM, Enjolras O, Mulliken JB. Congenital hemangioma: evidence of accelerated involution. J Pediatr 1996;128:329–35.

[51] Enjolras O, Mulliken JB, Boon LM, et al. Noninvoluting congenital hemangioma: a rare cutaneous vascular anomaly. Plast Reconstr Surg 2001; 107:1647–54.

[52] Waner M, North PE, Scherer KA, et al. The nonrandom distribution of facial hemangiomas. Arch Dermatol 2003;139:869–75.

[53] Metry DW, Dowd CF, Barkovich AJ, et al. The many faces of PHACE syndrome. J Pediatr 2001;139:117–23.

[54] Metry DW, Hawrot A, Altman C, et al. Association of solitary, segmental hemangiomas of the skin with visceral hemangiomatosis. Arch Dermatol 2004;140:591–6.

[55] Bronzetti G, Giardini A, Patrizi A, et al. Ipsilateral hemangioma and aortic arch anomalies in posterior fossa malformations, hemangiomas, arterial anomalies, coarctation of the aorta, and cardiac defects and eye abnormalities (PHACE) anomaly: report and review. Pediatrics 2004; 113:412–5.

[56] Coats DK, Paysse EA, Levy ML. PHACE: a neurocutaneous syndrome with important ophthalmologic implications: case report and literature review. Ophthalmology 1999;106:1739–41.

NEUROIMAGING
CLINICS
OF NORTH AMERICA

Neuroimag Clin N Am 17 (2007) 259–267

ELSEVIER
SAUNDERS

Pediatric Neuroanesthesia

Sulpicio G. Soriano, MD*, Elizabeth A. Eldredge, MD,
Mark A. Rockoff, MD

Recent advances in pediatric neurosurgery have dramatically improved the outcome in infants and children afflicted with surgical lesions of the central nervous system (CNS). Although most of these techniques were first applied to adults, the physiologic and developmental differences that are inherent in pediatric patients present challenges to neurosurgeons and anesthesiologists alike. The aim of this paper is to highlight these age-dependent approaches to the pediatric neurosurgical patient.

Developmental considerations

Age-dependent differences in cerebrovascular physiology and cranial bone development influence the approach to the pediatric neurosurgical patient. Cerebral blood flow is coupled tightly to metabolic demand, and both increase proportionally immediately after birth. Estimates from animal studies place the autoregulatory range of blood pressure in a normal newborn between 20 and 60 mmHg [1]. This range is consistent with relatively low cerebral metabolic requirements and low blood pressure during the perinatal period. More importantly, the slope of the autoregulatory slope drops and rises significantly at the lower and upper limits of the curve, respectively. This narrow range, with sudden hypotension and hypertension at either end of the autoregulatory curve, places the neonate at risk for cerebral ischemia and intraventricular hemorrhage, respectively. Another developmental difference between adults and pediatric patients is the larger percentage of cardiac output that is directed to the brain, because the head of the infant and child accounts for a large percentage of the body surface area and blood volume. These factors place the infant at risk for significant hemodynamic instability during neurosurgical procedures.

The infant cranial vault is also in a state of flux. Open fontanels and cranial sutures lead to a compliant intracranial space. The mass effect of a tumor or hemorrhage are often masked by a compensatory increase in the intracranial volume through the fontanels and sutures. As a result, infants presenting

---

This article has been previously published in Anesthesia Clinics.
Children's Hospital and Harvard Medical School, 300 Longwood Avenue, Boston, MA 02115, USA
* Corresponding author.
E-mail address: sulpicio.soriano@tch.harvard.edu (S.G. Soriano).

doi:10.1016/j.nic.2007.03.010

with signs and symptoms of intracranial hypertension have fairly advanced pathology.

Preoperative evaluation and preparation

Closed-claim studies have revealed that neonates and infants are at higher risk for morbidity and mortality than any other age group [2,3]. Respiratory and cardiac-related events account for a majority of these complications. However, a major pitfall in the management of infants and children for neurosurgery is the presence of coexisting diseases. Given the urgent nature of most pediatric neurosurgical procedures, a thorough preoperative evaluation may be difficult. However, a complete airway examination is essential, because some craniofacial anomalies may require specialized techniques to secure the airway [4]. Most cardiac morbidity due to congenital heart disease occurs during the first year of life [5]. Congenital heart disease may not be apparent immediately after birth, and the hemodynamic alterations caused by anesthetic agents, mechanical ventilation, and blood loss during surgery can unmask these cardiac defects. Echocardiography can be helpful in the assessment of the heart, and a pediatric cardiologist should evaluate patients with suspected problems to help optimize cardiac function prior to surgery. Other coexisting diseases that can alter the conduct of anesthesia are list in Table 1.

Preoperative sedatives given prior to induction of anesthesia can ease the transition from the preoperative holding area to the operating room [6]. Midazolam given orally is particularly effective in relieving anxiety and producing amnesia. If an indwelling intravenous (i.v.) catheter is in place, midazolam can be slowly administered to achieve sedation. Alternatively, sedatives such as barbiturates can be given rectally to induce sleep in preschool children who are uncooperative, and this avoids the use of intramuscular injections. However, methohexital administered rectally has been shown to induce seizures in patients with epilepsy [7].

Intraoperative management

Induction of anesthesia

The patient's neurological status and coexisting abnormalities will dictate the appropriate technique and drugs for induction of anesthesia. General anesthesia can be established by inhalation of sevoflurane and nitrous oxide with oxygen. A nondepolarizing muscle relaxant such as pancuronium is then administered to facilitate intubation of the trachea. Alternatively, if the patient has i.v. access, anesthesia can be rapidly induced with sedative/hypnotic drugs such thiopental (5–8 mg/kg)

or propofol (3–5 mg/kg). Patients at risk for aspiration pneumonitis should have a rapid-sequence induction of anesthesia performed with thiopental or propofol, immediately followed by a rapid-acting muscle relaxant such as succinylcholine or rocuronium.

Airway management

Developmental differences in the cricothyroid and tracheobronchial tree have a significant impact on management of the pediatric airway. The infant's larynx is funnel shaped, and narrowest at the level of the cricoid, making this the smallest cross-sectional area in the infant airway. This feature places the infant at risk for subglottic obstruction secondary to mucosal swelling after prolonged endotracheal intubation with a tight-fitting endotracheal tube. Because the trachea is relatively short, an endotracheal tube can migrate into a mainstem bronchus if the infant's head is flexed, as is the case for a suboccipital approach to the posterior

Table 1: Perioperative concerns for infants and children with neurological disease

Condition	Anesthetic implications
Congenital heart disease	Hypoxia and cardiovascular collapse
Prematurity	Postoperative apnea
Upper respiratory tract infection	Laryngospasm and postoperative hypoxia/pneumonia
Craniofacial abnormality	Difficulty with airway management
Denervation injuries	Hyperkalemia after succinycholine Resistance to nondepolarizing muscle relaxants
Chronic anticonvulsant therapy for epilepsy	Hepatic and hematological abnormalities Increased metabolism of anesthetic agents
Arteriovenous malformation	Potential congestive heart failure
Neuromuscular disease	Malignant hyperthermia Respiratory failure Sudden cardiac death
Chiari malformation	Apnea Aspiration pneumonitis
Hypothalamic/pituitary lesions	Diabetes insipidus Hypothyroidism Adrenal insufficiency

fossa or the cervical spine. Therefore, the anesthesiologist should auscultate both lung fields to rule out inadvertent intubation of a mainstem bronchus after positioning the patient. Nasotracheal tubes are best suited for situations when the patient will be prone and when postoperative mechanical ventilation is anticipated. Furthermore, the endotracheal tube can kink at the base of the tongue when the head is flexed and also lead to pressure necrosis of the oral mucosa.

Maintenance of anesthesia

The choice of anesthetic agents for maintenance of anesthesia has been shown not to affect the outcome of neurosurgical procedures [8]. The most frequently utilized technique for neurosurgery consists of the opioid fentanyl administered at a rate of 2–5 µg/kg/h intravenously along with inhaled nitrous oxide (70%) and low-dose isoflurane (0.2–0.5%). Deep neuromuscular blockade is maintained during most neurosurgical procedures to avoid patient movement. Patients on chronic anticonvulsant therapy will require larger doses of muscle relaxants and narcotics because of induced enzymatic metabolism of these agents (Fig. 1) [9,10]. Muscle relaxation should be withheld, or should not be maintained, when assessment of motor function during seizure and spinal cord surgery is planned.

Fluid restriction and diuretic therapy may lead to hemodynamic instability and even cardiovascular collapse if sudden blood loss occurs during surgery. Therefore, normovolemia should be maintained through the procedure. Normal saline is commonly used as the maintenance fluid during neurosurgery because it is mildly hyperosmolar (308 mOsm/kg), and it theoretically attenuates brain edema. However, rapid infusion of normal saline (30 mL/kg/h) is associated with hyperchloremic acidosis [11]. Hyperventilation and maximization of venous drainage of the brain by elevating the head can minimize brain swelling. Should these maneuvers fail, mannitol can be given at a dose of 0.25 to 1.0 g/kg intravenously. This will transiently alter cerebral hemodynamics and raise serum osmolality by 10–20 mOsm/kg [12]. However, repeated dosing can lead to extreme hyperosmolality, renal failure, and further brain edema. Furosemide is a useful adjunct to mannitol in decreasing acute cerebral edema and has been shown in vitro to prevent rebound swelling due to mannitol [13]. All diuretics will interfere with the ability to utilize urine output as a guide to intravascular volume status.

Vascular access

Due to limited access to the child during neurosurgical procedures, optimal intravenous access is mandatory prior to the start of surgery. Typically, two large-bore venous cannulae are sufficient for

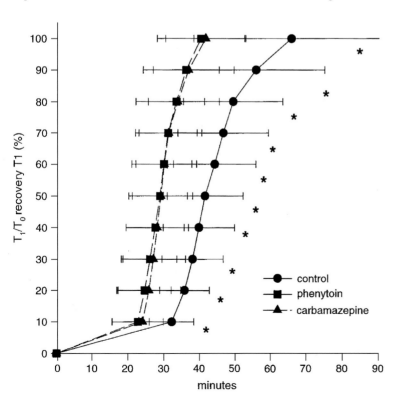

Fig. 1. Patients on chronic anticonvulsant therapy have increased requirements for nondepolarizing muscle relaxants. The recovery times for return of muscle function in the anticonvulsant group was significantly faster than the control group (*p < 0.05, mean ± SD). (*Adapted from* Soriano SG, Sullivan LJ, Venkatakrishnan K, et al. Pharmacokinetics and pharmacodynamics of vecuronium in children recieving phenytoin or carbamazepine for chronic anticonvulsant therapy. Br J Anaesth 2001;86:227; with permission.)

most craniotomies. Should initial attempts fail, central vein cannulation may be necessary. Cannulation of a femoral vein avoids the risk of pneumothorax associated with subclavian catheters and does not interfere with cerebral venous return.

Monitoring

Given the potential for sudden hemodynamic instability due to venous air emboli (VAE), hemorrhage, herniation syndromes, and manipulation of cranial nerves, the placement of an intra-arterial cannula for continuous blood pressure monitoring is mandatory for most neurosurgical procedures. An arterial catheter will also provide access for sampling serial blood gases, electrolytes, and hematocrit. The issue of central venous catheterization is controversial. Large-bore catheters are too large for infants and most children, and central venous pressures may not accurately reflect vascular volume, especially in a child in the prone position. Therefore, the risks may outweigh the benefits of a central venous catheter.

Standard neurosurgical technique may elevate the head of the table to improve venous drainage and is conducive to air entrainment into the venous system through open venous channels in bone and sinuses (Fig. 2) [14]. Patients with cardiac defects, such as patent foramen ovale or ductus arteriosus, are at risk for arterial air emboli through these defects, and should be monitored carefully. A precordial Doppler ultrasound can detect minute VAE and should be routinely used in conjunction with an end-tidal carbon dioxide analyzer and arterial catheter in all craniotomies to detect VAE. A Doppler probe is best positioned on the anterior chest usually just to the right of the sternum at the fourth intercostal space. An alternate site on the posterior thorax can be used in infants weighing approximately 6 kg or less [15].

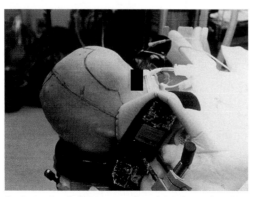

Fig. 2. Supine infant. Note that the infant's head lies at a higher plane than the rest of his body. This increases the likelihood for venous air embolism during craniotomies.

Recent advances in neurophysiologic monitoring have enhanced the ability to safely perform more definitive neurosurgical resections in functional areas of the brain and spinal cord. However, the CNS depressant effects of most anesthetic agents limit the utility of these monitors. A major part of preoperative planning should include a thorough discussion of the modality and type of neurophysiologic monitoring to be used during any surgical procedure. In general, electro-corticography (ECoG) and electroencephalography (EEG) require low levels of volatile anesthetics and barbiturates. Somatosensory-evoked potentials used during spinal and brainstem surgery can be depressed by volatile agents and to a lesser extent, nitrous oxide. An opioid-based anesthetic is the most appropriate agent for this type of monitoring. Spinal cord and peripheral nerve surgery may require electromyography (EMG) and detection of muscle movement as an end point. Therefore, muscle relaxation should be avoided or not maintained during the monitoring period.

Positioning

Patient positioning for surgery requires careful preoperative planning to allow adequate access to the patient for both the neurosurgeon and anesthesiologist. Table 2 describes various surgical positions and their physiologic sequelae. The prone position is commonly used for posterior fossa and spinal cord surgery, although the sitting position may be more appropriate for obese patients who may be difficult to ventilate in the prone position (Fig. 3). In addition to the physiologic sequelae of this position, a whole spectrum of compression and stretch injuries has been reported. Padding under the chest and pelvis can support the torso. It is important to ensure free abdominal wall motion because increased intra-abdominal pressure can impair ventilation, cause venocaval compression, and increase epidural venous pressure and bleeding. Fig. 4 illustrates proper positioning for these patients. Soft rolls are used to elevate and support the lateral chest wall and hips to minimize increase abdominal and thoracic pressure. In addition, this should allow a Doppler probe to be on the chest without pressure. Many neurosurgical procedures are performed with the head slightly elevated to facilitate venous and cerebral spinal fluid (CSF) drainage from the surgical site. However, superior sagittal sinus pressure decreases with increasing head elevation, and this increases the likelihood of VAE [14].

Extreme head flexion can cause brainstem compression in patients with posterior fossa pathology, such as mass lesions or an Arnold-Chiari malformation. Extreme rotation of the head can impede venous return through the jugular veins and lead to

Table 2: Physiologic effects of patient positioning

Position	Physiological effect
Head-elevated	Enhanced cerebral venous drainage
	Decreased cerebral blood flow
	Increased venous pooling in lower extremities
	Postural hypotension
Head-down	Increased cerebral venous and intracranial pressure
	Decreased functional residual capacity (lung function)
	Decreased lung compliance
Prone	Venous congestion of face, tongue, and neck
	Decreased lung compliance
	Increased abdominal pressure can lead to venocaval compression
Lateral decubitus	Decreased compliance of down-side lung

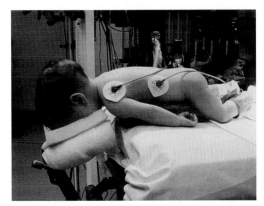

Fig. 4. Prone infant. Lateral rolls are used to elevate the infant and minimize thoracic and abdominal pressure.

impaired cerebral perfusion, increased intracranial pressure, and cerebral venous bleeding.

Postoperative management

Close observation in an intensive care unit with serial neurologic examinations and invasive hemodynamic monitoring is helpful for the prevention and early detection of postoperative problems. Respiratory dysfunction is the leading complication after posterior fossa craniotomies [16]. Airway edema is usually self-limited and may require endotracheal intubation as a stent. Occasionally, ischemia or edema of the respiratory centers in the brainstem will interfere with respiratory control and lead to postoperative apnea. Children with Chiari malformations may be more prone to the respiratory depression [17]. Diabetes insipidus can occur after surgery in the region of the hypothalamus and pituitary gland, and can be managed acutely with an intravenous vasopressin infusion. Postoperative nausea and vomiting can cause sudden rises in intracranial pressure and should be treated with a nonsedating antiemetic. However, prophylactic administration of ondansteron during surgery is not effective in decreasing the incidence of vomiting following craniotomies in children [18].

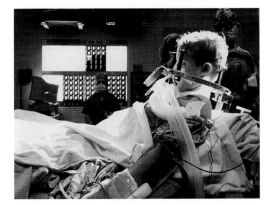

Fig. 3. Sitting position. The sitting position affords optimal chest wall compliance in children with respiratory disease and obesity.

Clinical approaches

Neonatal emergencies

Most neonatal surgery is performed on an emergent basis [19], and there is more than a 10-fold increase in perioperative morbidity and mortality in neonates when compared with other pediatric age groups [2]. In addition to existing congenital heart defects, congestive heart failure can occur in neonates with large cerebral arteriovenous malformations, and this condition requires aggressive hemodynamic support. Management of the neonatal respiratory system may be difficult because of the diminutive size of the airway, craniofacial anomalies, laryngotracheal lesions, and acute (hyaline membrane disease, retained amniotic fluid) or chronic (bronchopulmonary dysplasia) disease. Because these conditions are in a state of flux, they should be addressed preoperatively to minimize morbidity.

The neonatal central nervous system is capable of sensing pain and mounting a stress response after a surgical stimulus [20]. However, neonatal myocardial function is particularly sensitive to both inhaled and intravenous anesthetics, and the use of these agents needs to be judicious to block surgical stress without causing myocardial depression. An opioid-based anesthetic is generally the most stable hemodynamic technique for neonates. The hepatic and renal systems are also not fully developed, and neonates anesthetized with a narcotic technique will often have delayed emergence and may require postoperative mechanical ventilation.

Closure of a myelomeningocele or encephalocele presents special problems. Positioning the patient for tracheal intubation may rupture the membranes covering the spinal cord or brain. Therefore, careful padding of the lesion (Fig. 5), and in some cases intubation of the neonate's trachea in the left lateral decubitus position, may be necessary. Most surgical closures of simple myelomeningoceles have relatively minimal blood loss. However, large lesions may requirement significant undermining of cutaneous tissue to cover the defect and pose larger risks for blood loss and hemodymanic instability. Recent advances in the management of myelomeningoceles have lead to early intervention into the

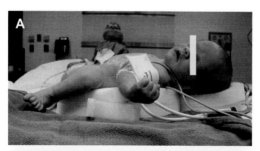

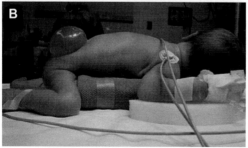

Fig. 5. Positioning of a neonate with a myelomeningocele. (*A*) Prior to induction of general anesthesia, the neonate is elevated on a soft padding with a center cutout to relieve pressure on the myelomeningocele. (*B*) Positioning of the neonate for closure of the myelomeningocele.

intrauterine period [21]. The management of the fetus and mother during fetal surgery has been reviewed extensively elsewhere [22,23].

Hydrocephalus

The most common neurosurgical procedure performed in major pediatric centers is for the management of hydrocephalus. Regardless of the etiology, whether it be overproduction of CSF due to choroid plexus papillomas or obstruction of CSF flow secondary to a tumor or Chiari malformation, diagnosis and alleviation of life-threatening intracranial hypertension should proceed expeditiously. The mental status of the child should dictate the anesthetic management as noted above, and intracranial hypertension can be managed with hyperventilation and diuretics. Most neonates undergoing a closure of a myelomeningocele are potential candidates for a ventriculo-peritoneal shunt (VPS) and may have both procedures performed in one sitting. The long-term management of hydrocephalus with VPS invariably increases the incidence of mechanical failure and shunt infections. Should the peritoneum be infected, alternate sites for the drainage limb of these extracranial shunts include the right atrium and pleural cavity.

Craniosynostosis

Repairs of craniosynostosis are likely to have the best result if done early in life [24]. However, these procedures are associated with loss of a significant percentage of an infant's blood volume, with great losses occurring when more sutures are involved [25]. Venous air embolism detected by echocardiography and precordial Doppler occurred in 66% to 83% of craniectomies in infants [25,26]. Fortunately, direct morbidity and mortality rarely occur. Venous air emboli can be minimized by early detection with continuous precordial Doppler ultrasound and maintaining euvolumia. When hemodynamic instability does occur, the operating table can be placed in the Trendelenburg position, flooding the surgical field with warm saline and sealing the sites of egress with bone wax and direct pressure. These maneuvers will augment the patient's blood pressure and prevent further entrainment of intravascular air.

Tumors

Because the majority of intracranial tumors in children occur in the posterior fossa, CSF flow is often obstructed, and intracranial hypertension and hydrocephalus is often present. Most neurosurgeons approach this region with children in the prone position. The patient's head is often secured with a Mayfield head frame. Pins used in small children can cause skull fractures, dural tears, and intracranial hematomas. Elevation of the bone flap can tear the transverse and straight sinuses, and massive blood loss and/or VAE can occur. Surgical resection of tumors in the posterior fossa can also lead to brainstem and/or cranial nerve damage. Sudden changes in blood pressure and heart rate may be sentinel signs of encroachment on these structures. Damage to the respiratory centers and cranial nerves can lead to apnea and airway obstruction after extubation of the patient's trachea. Children requiring stereotactic-guided radiosurgery or craniotomies need general anesthesia to tolerate the procedures. Special head frames have been devised to allow airway manipulations and should be used in these patients [27].

Epilepsy

Surgical treatment has become a viable option for many patients with medically intractable epilepsy. Two major considerations should be kept in mind. Chronic administration of anticonvulsant drugs, phenytoin and carbamazepine, induces rapid metabolism and clearance of several classes of anesthetic agents including neuromuscular blockers and opioids [9,28]. Therefore, the anesthetic requirements for these drugs are increased and require close monitoring of their effect and frequent redosing. Intraoperative neurophysiologic monitors can be used to guide the actual resection of the epileptogenic focus, and general anesthetics can compromise the sensitivity of these devices [29].

Because some epileptogenic foci are in close proximity to cortical areas controlling speech, memory, and motor or sensory function, monitoring of patient and electrophysiologic responses are frequently utilized to minimize iatrogenic injury to these areas [30,31]. Cortical stimulation of the motor strip in a child under general anesthesia will require either EMG or direct visualization of muscle movement. Neuromuscular blockade should not be used in this situation. Neural function is best assessed in an awake and cooperative patient. Awake craniotomies in children can be accomplished with local anesthesia and propofol and fentanyl for sedation and analgesia, respectively [32]. Positioning of the patient is critical for success of this technique. The patient should be in a semilateral position to allow both patient comfort as well as surgical and airway access to the patient. Propofol does not interfere with the ECoG if it is discontinued 20 minutes before monitoring. Highly motivated children older that 10 years of age were able to withstand the procedure without incident. However, it is imperative that candidates for an awake craniotomy be mature and psychologically prepared to participate in this procedure. Therefore, patients who are developmentally delayed or have a history of severe anxiety or psychiatric disorders should not be considered appropriate for an awake craniotomy. Very young patients cannot be expected to cooperate for these procedures and usually require general anesthesia with extensive neurophysiologic monitoring to minimize inadvertent resection of the motor strip and eloquent cortex. Repeat craniotomies for removal of ECoG leads and depth electrodes used for chronic invasive EEG monitoring and subsequent resection of the seizure focus are at risk for expansion of residual pneumocephalus. It is important to avoid nitrous oxide until the dura is opened, because intracranial air can persist up to 3 weeks following a craniotomy [33].

Vascular

Vascular anomalies are rare in infants and children. Most of these conditions are congenital anomalies and present early in life. Large arteriovenous malformations (AVM) in neonates may be associated with high output congestive heart failure and require vasoactive support. Initial treatment of large AVMs often consists of intravascular embolization in the radiologic suite [34]. Operative management is commonly associated with massive blood loss, and these patients require several i.v. access sites and invasive hemodynamic monitoring. Ligation of an AVM can lead to sudden hypertension with hyperemic cerebral edema [35]. Vasodilators such as labetalol or nitroprusside can be used to control a hypertensive crisis.

Moyamoya syndrome is a rare chronic vaso-occlusive disorder of the internal carotid arteries that presents as transient ischemic attacks and/or recurrent strokes in childhood. The etiology is unknown, but the syndrome can be associated with prior intracranial radiation, neurofibromatosis, Down's syndrome, and a variety of hematological disorders. The anesthetic management of these patients is directed at optimizing cerebral perfusion by maintaining euvolemia and the blood pressure within the patient's preoperative levels [36]. Maintenance of normocapnia is also essential in patients with Moyamoya syndrome because both hyper- and hypocapnia can lead to stealing phenomenon from the ischemic region and further aggravate cerebral ischemia [37]. A nitrous oxide and narcotic-based anesthetic provides a stable level of anesthesia for these patients, and is compatible with intraoperative EEG monitoring. Once the patient emerges from anesthesia, the same maneuvers that optimize cerebral perfusion should be extended into the postoperative period. These patients should receive i.v. fluids to maintain adequate cerebral perfusion and be given adequate narcotics to avoid hyperventilation induced by pain and crying.

Trauma

Pediatric head trauma requires a multiorgan approach to minimizing morbidity and mortality [38]. A small child's head is often the point of impact in injuries, but other organs can also be damaged. Basic life support algorithms should be immediately applied to assure a patent airway, spontaneous respiration, and adequate circulation. Immobilization of the cervical spine is essential to avoid secondary injury with manipulation of the patient's airway until radiologic clearance is confirmed. Blunt abdominal trauma and long bone fractures frequently occur with head injury and can be major sources of blood loss. To assure tissue perfusion during the operative period, the patient's blood volume should be restored with crystalloid solutions and/or blood products. Ongoing blood loss can lead to coagulopathies and should be treated with specific blood components.

Infants with "Shaken Baby Syndrome" often present with a myriad of chronic and acute subdural hematomas [39]. As with all traumatic events, the presence of other coexisting injuries, fractures, and abdominal trauma should be identified. Craniotomies for the evacuation of either epidural or subdural hematomas are at high risk for massive blood loss and VAE. Postoperative management of these victims is marked by the management of intracranial hypertension and, in the most severe cases, determination of brain death.

Spine surgery

Spinal dysraphism is the primary indication for laminectomies in pediatric patients. Many of these patients have a history of a meningomyelocele closure followed by several corrective surgeries. These patients have been exposed to latex products and may develop hypersensitivity to latex. Latex allergy can manifest itself by a severe anaphylactic reaction heralded by hypotension and wheezing, and should be rapidly treated by removal of the source of latex and administration of fluid and vasopressors [40]. Patients at risk for latex allergy should have a latex-free environment.

Tethered cord releases require EMG monitoring to help identify functional nerve roots. EMG of the anal sphincter and muscles of the lower extremities is performed intraoperatively to minimize inadvertent injury to nerves innervating these muscle groups [41]. Muscle relaxation should be discontinued or antagonized to allow accurate EMG monitoring.

Neuroradiology

Recent advances in imaging technology have provided less invasive procedures to diagnose and treat lesions in the CNS. Most neuroradiological studies such as CT scans and magnetic resonance imaging can be accomplished with light sedation. Recommendations have been published by consensus groups of anesthesiologists and pediatricians, and can serve as guidelines for managing these patients [42,43]. General anesthesia is typically used for uncooperative patients, patients with coexisting medical problems, and potentially painful procedures such as intravascular embolization of vascular lesions [34].

Summary

The perioperative management of pediatric neurosurgical patients presents many challenges to neurosurgeons and anesthesiologists. Many conditions are unique to pediatrics. Thorough preoperative evaluation and open communication between members of the health care team are important. A basic understanding of age-dependent variables and the interaction of anesthetic and surgical procedures are essential in minimizing perioperative morbidity and mortality.

References

[1] Pryds O. Control of cerebral circulation in the high-risk neonate. Ann Neurol 1991;30:321–9.
[2] Cohen MM, Cameron CB, Duncan PG. Pediatric anesthesia morbidity and mortality in the perioperative period. Anesth Analg 1990;70:160–7.
[3] Morray JP, Geiduschek JM, Ramamoorthy C, et al. Anesthesia-related cardiac arrest in children: initial findings of the Pediatric Perioperative Cardiac Arrest (POCA) Registry. Anesthesiology 2000;93:6–14.
[4] Nargozian CD. The difficult airway in the pediatric patient with craniofacial anomaly. Anesthesiol Clin North Am 1999;16:839–52.
[5] Boneva RS, Botto LD, Moore CA, Yang Q, Correa A, Erickson JD. Mortality associated with congenital heart defects in the United States: trends and racial disparities, 1979–1997. Circulation 2001;103:2376–81.
[6] McCann ME, Kain ZN. Management of perioperative anxiety in children. Anesth Analg 2001;93:98–105.
[7] Rockoff MA, Goudsouzian NG. Seizures induced by methohexital. Anesthesiology 1981;54:333–5.
[8] Todd MM, Warner DS, Sokoll MD, et al. A prospective, comparative trial of three anesthetics for elective supratentorial craniotomy. Anesthesiology 1993;78:1005–20.
[9] Soriano SG, Kaus SJ, Sullivan LJ, et al. Onset and duration of action of rocuronium in children receiving chronic anticonvulsant therapy. Paediatr Anaesth 2000;10:133–6.
[10] Soriano SG, Sullivan LJ, Venkatakrishnan K, et al. Pharmacokinetics and pharmacodynamics of vecuronium in children receiving phenytoin or

carbamazepine for chronic anticonvulsant therapy. Br J Anaesth 2001;86:223–9.

[11] Scheingraber S, Rehm M, Sehmisch C, et al. Rapid saline infusion produces hyperchloremic acidosis in patients undergoing gynecologic surgery. Anesthesiology 1999;90:1265–70.

[12] Soriano SG, McManus ML, Sullivan LJ, et al. Cerebral blood flow velocity after mannitol infusion in children. Can J Anaesth 1996;43:461–6.

[13] McManus ML, Soriano SG. Rebound swelling of astroglial cells exposed to hypertonic mannitol. Anesthesiology 1998;88:1586–91.

[14] Grady MS, Bedford RF, Park TS. Changes in superior sagittal sinus pressure in children with head elevation, jugular venous compression, and PEEP. J Neurosurg 1986;65:199–202.

[15] Soriano SG, McManus ML, Sullivan LJ, et al. Doppler sensor placement during neurosurgical procedures for children in the prone position. J Neurosurg Anesthesiol 1994;6:153–5.

[16] Meridy HW, Creighton RE, Humphreys RB. Complications during neurosurgical procedures in the prone position. Can J Anaesth 1974;21:445–52.

[17] Waters KA, Forbes P, Morielli A, et al. Sleep-disordered breathing in children with myelomeningocele. J Pediatr 1998;132:672–81.

[18] Furst SR, Sullivan LJ, Soriano SG, et al. Effects of ondansetron on emesis in the first 24 hours after craniotomy in children. Anesth Analg 1996;83:325–8.

[19] Koka BV, Soriano SG. Anesthesia for neonatal surgical emergencies. Semin Anesthes 1992;9:309–16.

[20] Anand KJ, Hickey PR. Pain and its effects in the human neonate and fetus. N Engl J Med 1987;317:1321–9.

[21] Sutton LN, Sun P, Adzick NS. Fetal neurosurgery. Neurosurgery 2001;48:124–42.

[22] Gaiser RR, Kurth CD. Anesthetic considerations for fetal surgery. Semin Perinatol 1999;23:507–14.

[23] O'Hara IB, Kurth CD. Anesthesia for fetal surgery. In: Greeley WJ, editor. Pediatric anesthesia. Philadelphia: Churchill Livingstone; 1999. p. 15.1–15.11.

[24] Shillito J Jr. A plea for early operation for craniosynostosis. Surg Neurol 1992;37:182–8.

[25] Faberowski LW, Black S, Mickle JP. Incidence of venous air embolism during craniectomy for craniosynostosis repair. Anesthesiology 2000;92:20–3.

[26] Harris MM, Yemen TA, Davidson A, et al. Venous embolism during craniectomy in supine infants. Anesthesiology 1987;67:816–9.

[27] Stokes MA, Soriano SG, Tarbell NJ, et al. Anesthesia for stereotactic radiosurgery in children. J Neurosurg Anesthesiol 1995;7:100–8.

[28] Tempelhoff R, Modica PA, Spitznagel EL. Anticonvulsants therapy increases fentanyl requirements during anaesthesia for craniotomy. Can J Anaesth 1990;37:327–32.

[29] Eldredge EA, Soriano SG, Rockoff MA. Neuroanesthesia. In: Adelson PD, Black PM, editors. Surgical treatment of epilepsy in children. Philadelphia: W.B. Saunders; 1995. p. 505–20.

[30] Black PM, Ronner SF. Cortical mapping for defining the limits of tumor resection. Neurosurgery 1987;20:914–9.

[31] Penfield W. Combined regional and general anesthesia for craniotomy and cortical exploration. Part I., Neurosurgical considerations. Anesth Analg 1954;33:145–55.

[32] Soriano SG, Eldredge EA, Wang FK, et al. The effect of propofol on intraoperative electro-corticography and cortical stimulation during awake craniotomies in children. Paediatr Anaesth 2000;10:29–34.

[33] Reasoner DK, Todd MM, Scamman FL, et al. The incidence of pneumocephalus after supratentorial craniotomy. Observations on the disappearance of intracranial air. Anesthesiology 1994;80:1008–12.

[34] Burrows PE, Robertson RL. Neonatal central nervous system vascular disorders. Neurosurg Clin North Am 1998;9:155–80.

[35] Morgan MK, Sekhon LH, Finfer S, et al. Delayed neurological deterioration following resection of arteriovenous malformations of the brain. J Neurosurg 1999;90:695–701.

[36] Soriano SG, Sethna NF, Scott RM. Anesthetic management of children with moyamoya syndrome. Anesth Analg 1993;77:1066–70.

[37] Kuwabara Y, Ichiya Y, Sasaki M, et al. Response to hypercapnia in moyamoya disease. Cerebrovascular response to hypercapnia in pediatric and adult patients with moyamoya disease. Stroke 1997;28:701–7.

[38] Lam WH, MacKersie A. Paediatric head injury: incidence, aetiology and management. Paediatr Anaesth 1999;9:377–85.

[39] Duhaime AC, Christian CW, Rorke LB, et al. Nonaccidental head injury in infants—the "shaken-baby syndrome". N Engl J Med 1998;338:1822–9.

[40] Holzman RS. Clinical management of latex-allergic children. Anesth Analg 1997;85:529–33.

[41] Legatt AD, Schroeder CE, Gill B, et al. Electrical stimulation and multichannel EMG recording for identification of functional neural tissue during cauda equina surgery. Childs Nerv Syst 1992;8:185–9.

[42] American Academy of Pediatrics Committee on Drugs. Guidelines for monitoring and management of pediatric patients during and after sedation for diagnostic and therapeutic procedures. Pediatrics 1992;89:1110–5.

[43] American Society of Anesthesiologists. Practice guidelines for sedation and analgesia by non-anesthesiologists. A report by the American Society of Anesthesiologists Task Force on Sedation and Analgesia by Non-Anesthesiologists. Anesthesiology 1996;84:459–71.

ELSEVIER
SAUNDERS

NEUROIMAGING
CLINICS
OF NORTH AMERICA

Neuroimag Clin N Am 17 (2007) 269–280

Overt and Incomplete (Silent) Cerebral Infarction in Sickle Cell Anemia: Diagnosis and Management

Wing-Yen Wong, MD[a], Darleen R. Powars, MD[b],*

- Risk factors
- Clinical diagnosis
- Neuroimaging
- Prevention
- Acute management

- Transfusion therapy
- Hydroxyurea
- Neurorehabilitation
- References

Cerebral vasculopathy in sickle cell anemia (HbSS) is manifest clinically as cerebral infarction and intracranial hemorrhage. The type of stroke, ischemic or hemorrhagic, is age specific with distinct differences in outcomes. Cerebral infarction with or without clinical stroke begins during early childhood and rarely causes death immediately [1,2]. Acute intracranial hemorrhage has been associated with high immediate mortality ranging from 24% to 50% [3–5].

The authors' overall calculated incidence of first overt infarction in HbSS patients by age 20 years is 11% and by age 45 years 24%. The highest frequency occurs in children aged 2 through 5 years followed by those aged 6 to 9 years. A second peak is observed in adults greater than 20 years of age (Fig. 1). The calculated median age of onset among the authors' subjects for clinically recognized cerebral infarctions is 13.88 years (range, 1.2 to 58.18) and for intracranial hemorrhage 31.75 years (range, 4.87 to 51.5 years).

The accumulative overall risk for cerebral infarction during the patient's lifetime, including clinical events and subclinical events, has been estimated to be as high as 30% [2,6,7]. This percentage rises even further if one uses improved MRI techniques, particularly fluid-attenuated inversion recovery (FLAIR) [8]. Steen and coworkers reported that 44% of patients demonstrated infarction, ischemia, or atrophy on MRI (FLAIR) and 49% had abnormal findings on MR angiography.

During the last decade, a changing prevalence pattern has been observed, with an increasing frequency of first identified clinical neurologic events at 20 to 25 years of age. Using definitive neuroimaging techniques based on the presence of areas of

This Article has been previously published in Hematology/Oncology Clinics.
[a] Department of Pediatrics, Division of Hematology/Oncology, Children's Hospital Los Angeles, Keck School of Medicine at the University of Southern California, Los Angeles, CA, USA
[b] Department of Pediatrics, Division of Hematology/Oncology, Women's & Children's Hospital, Keck School of Medicine at the University of Southern California, 1240 North Mission Road, Room L902, Los Angeles, CA 90033, USA
* Corresponding author.
E-mail address: powars@hsc.usc.edu (D.R. Powars).

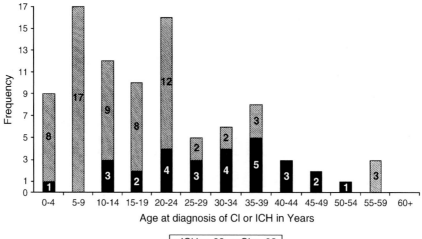

Fig. 1. Age and type of first cerebral vascular accident in hemoglobin SS subjects. The specific type of clinical stroke was identified based on neuroimaging or autopsy in 91 subjects with sickle cell anemia. Intracranial hemorrhage (ICH) was found in 28 subjects and cerebral infarction (CI) in 63. Six subjects not shown on the figure had CI followed by ICH, and 23 subjects had an unspecified CVA usually occurring before contemporary neuroimaging capability was available (N = 122).

cerebral atrophy or old infarcts in the border zone regions, it is clear that these patients have "silent" stroke (incomplete infarctions) [9] before overt clinical stroke becomes apparent [10]. The overall prevalence of stroke including cerebral infarction and intracranial hemorrhage is close to reaching the level observed in children between 2 and 9 years of age. The clinical demarcation line is blurring between overt stroke and incomplete infarction, particularly during the third decade of life. This phenomenon is most obvious in the patients who the authors observed during the calendar era of 1980 through 1995 as children. At that time, these patients had evidence of incomplete infarctions based on positron-emission tomography (PET) technology [11] but were not placed on transfusion therapy or hydroxyurea. They now appear with identified neurologic events during the third decade life.

Risk factors

Clinical and laboratory risk factors for cerebral infarction are listed in Box 1 [3,12–16]. Seventeen percent of North American HbSS children who had three or more risk factors by age 2 years demonstrated a 38.3% frequency of subsequent clinical stroke by age 8 years [17]. In a prospective study, Glauser and coworkers observed the onset of a first neurologic event between 2.4 and 6.1 years in children who had a transient ischemic attack (TIA) or effervescent neurologic symptoms. These children had incomplete infarction (silent) at a rate of 71%

(12 of 17) on conventional MRI. Wang and coworkers [19] showed that 7 of 39 very young neurologically asymptomatic children had significant magnetic resonance neuroimaging abnormalities. Border zone silent infarction combined with elevated blood flow velocity on Doppler analysis increased the risk of overt clinical stroke [20]. Recently, Steen and Ogg [16] have demonstrated that HbSS children have elevated brain N-acetylaspartate, a highly specific marker for neurons. Normal glial cells express a high-affinity for N-acetylaspartate [15]. The transport into glial cells is obligatory for myelination and repair. No risk factor analysis can distinguish between the patient who will progress to clinical stroke and the patient who will sustain slowly enlarging penumbral ischemia or new incomplete infarctions. Border zone infarctions in adults that are identified during childhood seem to be a risk factor for subsequent infarction and intracranial hemorrhage. The observation that the acute chest syndrome rate and recurrence during young childhood is a risk factor for clinical stroke [21] seems to carry over as a comorbid predictor in adult patients with developing chronic pulmonary disease. Systolic hypertension, which is frequently associated with adult onset uremia, is a significant risk factor for intracranial hemorrhage.

Using the criteria in Box 1, a high-risk HbSS child should be evaluated at 3 years of age. The neuroimaging evaluation should include ultrasonography of the branches of the internal carotid arteries (ICA), distal carotid siphon (dICA), middle cerebral artery (MCA), and anterior cerebral artery

Box 1: Cerebral infarction: factors predictive of risk

Clinical Factors
- Age 2 through 8 years (elevated cerebral flood flow)
- HbSS sibling with stroke
- Incomplete (silent) infarction
- Prior TIA
- Bacterial meningitis
- B19 infection–induced aplastic crisis
- Repeat episodes of severe acute chest syndrome with hypoxia (PaO$_2$) <60 mm Hg
- Nocturnal hypoxemia with or without sleep apnea
- Acute anemic episode (Hb 2 g/dL below normal level)
- Repeat seizure episodes
- Dactylitis before age 1 year
- Splenic dysfunction or infarction near age 1 year
- Priapism
- Systolic hypertension[a]
- Decreasing academic school performance
- Decreasing fine motor skills (Zurick fine motor examination, Perdue non-dominant hand pegboard)
- Abnormal test of variables of attention

Laboratory Risk Factors
- Hemoglobin (steady state) concentration <7.5 g/dL with high reticulocyte count
- Leukocyte count >15 × 10^9/L
- Platelet count >450 × 10^9/L
- Pocked (pitted) red blood cells ≥3.5% by 24 months of age
- Fetal hemoglobin ≤13% by age 24 months
- No alpha gene deletion [14]
- HLA subtypes (DPBI*0401)
- HLA-A*0102, HLA-A*2612 [13]

Observations in young children during steady state, not recently transfused, and not on chemotherapy (hydroxyurea) [3,12–16]. In a prospective natural history study. For the 17% of North American HbSS children who had three or more risk factors by age 2 years, the frequency of clinical stroke by age 8 years was 38.3% [17].
[a] Frequently associated with adult onset uremia and intracranial hemorrhage.

(ACA) (Fig. 2). This evaluation should be followed by diffusion-weighted (DWI) or FLAIR MRI and MR angiography [22]. Abnormalities seen on this combination of studies increase the subsequent infarction risk to greater than 50% in the untreated child [1,23]. The identification of dICA and MCA stenosis, conventional MRI border zone lesions, and loss of gray matter on quantitative or FLAIR MRI is evidence of disease progression. Cognitive deficiency may be inevitable [24], although overt stroke and severe cognitive disability should be preventable with adequate treatment [25].

Clinical diagnosis

Clinical diagnosis of cerebral infarction with overt hemiparesis and hemisensory loss is not difficult [6,26–28]. More difficult is the diagnosis of less overt dysfunction such as the weakness of one leg or arm. TIAs are not frequently recognized during childhood and adolescence. The reason for this may be the subtleness of the findings and the transient nature of a mild hemiparesis of less than 24 hours. The problem of nonrecognition of mild stroke symptomatology or TIA has been reported in a group of children with and without sickle cell disease. Gabis and coworkers [29] identified that, in children, the time from clinical onset to first medical contact averaged 28.5 hours and the time to diagnosis 35.7 hours. Remarkably, young patients are often not taken to the physician who is aware of the risk of stroke. The patient's family becomes accustomed to pain in the child's arms and legs and often states that they thought the weakness of an extremity was secondary to a pain crisis [30].

The most important aspect of the physical examination at age 3 years during risk assessment is observing the child walking, jumping, standing on one leg, and playing. Any uneven gait or inability to use both hands and arms when placing one block upon another should heighten the sense that this child may already have had an incomplete infarction and should act as a impetus for rapid neurodiagnostic testing [18].

The association of incomplete (silent) infarction on conventional MRI with an increase in subsequent clinical stroke and cognitive dysfunction has been documented in children [20,31–35] and seems to be present in young adults. The progressive accumulation of incomplete neurovascular infarcts leads to poorer intellectual function.

The combined application of anatomic and physiologic neuroimaging modalities in high-risk young HbSS children can improve the predictive accuracy of impending stroke during the first decade of life [36,37]. Neuroimaging border zone abnormalities without a complete infarction combined with the finding of elevated velocity on ultrasonography define a "window of opportunity" that should prompt the initiation of preventative therapy before the development and diagnosis of overt stroke [1]. Fifty-two percent (52%) of children with border zone abnormalities combined with elevated transcranial Doppler ultrasonography experienced new or expanded silent (incomplete) infarctions or overt stroke. Cognitive disability is a major consequence of microvascular ischemia even without overt

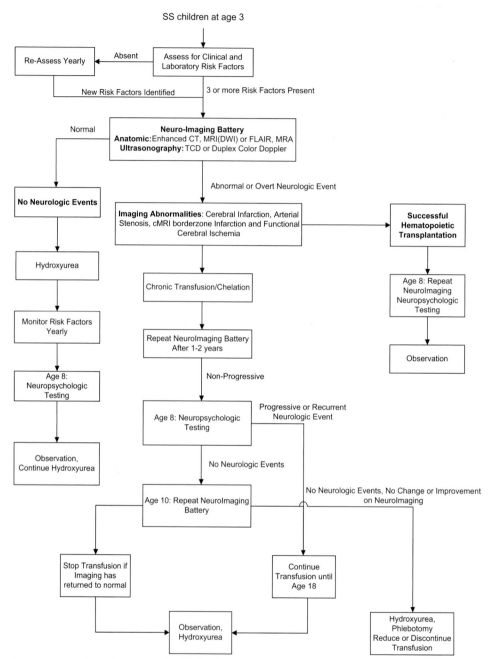

Fig. 2. Management algorithm for cerebral infarction in children with sickle cell anemia. Clinical and laboratory risk factors are listed in **Box 1**. cMRI, conventional MRI; CT, computed tomography; FLAIR, fluid-attenuated inversion recovery MRI; MRA, MR angiography; MRI (DWI), diffusion-weighted MRI; TCD, ultrasonography using transcranial Doppler.

clinical stroke [38]. Falling off neurodevelopmental milestones is an indicator for further neuropsychologic evaluation and diagnosis.

Beyond the third decade, intracranial hemorrhage is the most common type of clinical stroke observed. After the third decade of life as end-stage renal disease and chronic lung disease with pulmonary hypertension increase in prevalence, these comorbidities enhance the risk of rupture of small fragile collateral vessels of the brain (Moyamoya like), which are often not recognized clinically to be present.

Neuroimaging

Essential to the diagnosis of cerebral vasculopathy in HbSS patients is the use of recently developed improvements in CT and MRI [35,39–42]. These imaging modalities confirm a clinical diagnosis of cerebral infarction in nearly 100% of HbSS subjects with hemiparetic hemisensory strokes. In addition, enhanced CT and the recently developed techniques of DWI and FLAIR MRI demonstrate exquisite detail about brain structure [43,44]. Cerebral infarction lesions appear hyperintense on T2-weighted conventional MRI images and are consistently associated with quantitative MRI (DWI) and FLAIR lesions in the contiguous penumbral cerebral lesions. Steen and coworkers [8] reported that FLAIR images demonstrated gray matter abnormalities present in 35% of HbSS subjects without known clinical stroke, similar to findings using PET technology [11,22]. Kirkham and coworkers [22] noted that perfusion abnormalities on DWI were larger than the conventional MRI infarction regions, identifying penumbral affected regions. FLAIR or DWI abnormalities are associated with soft neurologic symptoms in patients with normal conventional MRI and normal ultrasonography velocities. It is now possible to perform anatomic studies rapidly using DWI or FLAIR images and MR angiography at one time using the same equipment with additional programming. This capability allows for a rapid assessment of the state of the cerebral vasculopathy, defining complete infarctions, incomplete infarctions, early gray matter neuronal loss without overt infarction, and the extent of the affected penumbral regions (Table 1). DWI detects acute ischemia when conventional MRI with spinecho T2-weighted images may still be normal and can be helpful in differentiating acute from chronic ischemic changes. In a small study, acute infarcts less than 6 hours old were detected correctly in only 18% of conventional MRI images, whereas all of the lesions were detected on DWI [40]. Comparison studies have shown equivalent specificity of MR angiography for the diagnosis of cerebral arterial stenosis when compared with conventional angiography or ultrasonography [37,45]. MR angiography can detect aneurysms of the circle of Willis and the narrow twisted fragile vessels characteristic of Moyamoya anomaly, which are prevalent in patients during the second, third, and fourth decades of life. Programming of T1-weighted MR angiography images can differentiate large vessel endothelial roughening with early stenosis from turbulent blood flow. Turbulence disappears after the anemia is corrected while stenosis of the major vessels remains evident. MR spectroscopy can detect significant metabolic changes in areas of recent ischemia, including the level of N-acetylaspartate. Increases in the level of lactate and glutamate and decreases in the level of N-acetylaspartate can be measured within minutes of the insult and are present for 3 to 6 hours. These acute changes are valuable in the differentiation of old infarction from new ischemic lesions in penumbral regions. In the old infarcts, readily seen on conventional MRI or enhanced CT scans, patients with stable neurologic deficits do not show specific spectral abnormalities.

Ultrasonography using transcranial Doppler or duplex color Doppler imaging provides a safe and noninvasive measure of blood flow velocity in the carotid siphon (dICA), proximal MCA, and proximal ACA [7]. The velocity of the posterior cerebral artery and basilar arteries is less well defined using transcranial Doppler imaging. The numeric velocities obtained by duplex color Doppler imaging are somewhat lower than those obtained by transcranial imaging. A velocity greater than 170 cm/s is diagnostic of significant stenosis on duplex Doppler imaging, whereas a velocity of 200 cm/s is the equivalent value on transcranial imaging [46]. Very high and very low velocities are manifestations of stenosis or incipient occlusions. Elevated blood flow velocities combined with MRI-detected incomplete infarction predict a significant risk of subsequent clinical stroke in HbSS children [1]. As HbSS patients are placed on transfusion therapy, the velocity in the MCA decreases [47].

The MRI appearance in infarction becomes more obvious in the subacute phase. The T1-weighted signal becomes more hypointense, and there are increases in the T2-weighted images making gray matter and white matter abnormalities more apparent. In HbSS patients, the most common sites of conventional MRI and CT abnormalities involve the frontal and parietal lobes. Brain atrophy is observed in approximately 20% of the patients on MRI and is better defined on enhanced CT scan.

CT reliably demonstrates nearly 100% of cases of acute parenchymal hemorrhage and subarachnoid hemorrhage. MRI is less reliable and variable. In a small study, FLAIR MRI had a sensitivity of 100% and was comparable with CT scans in the detection of acute intracranial hemorrhage [48]. On FLAIR images, the signal of normal cerebrospinal fluid is suppressed; therefore, the signal intensity of hemorrhage is higher than that of cerebrospinal fluid and the surrounding gray matter. When possible, the physician responsible for clinical case management should request DWI or FLAIR MRI for infarction and enhanced CT for hemorrhage in the diagnostic neuroimaging of these subjects.

Table 1: **Brain imaging modalities**

Modality	Physiologic activity	Advantages	Disadvantages
Transcranial Doppler ultrasonography (TCD)	Measures elevated blood flow velocity in dICA, MCA, ACA >200 cm/s in anemic children	Portable Best used for screening of presymptomatic cerebrovascular disease	Nonduplex (no direct visualization of vessels) Cannot demonstrate small vessel disease Requires special training Velocity decreases to normal in transfused subjects
Modifications of color duplex Doppler ultrasonography including high-resolution B-mode ultrasonography	Measures cerebral blood vessel flow Measures cerebral vessel intima/media thickness >170 cm/s in anemic children is conditionally elevated	Direct duplex visualization of cerebral vessels Good visualization of bifurcation of distal internal carotid artery, posterior cerebral artery, basilar artery Best used for screening for cerebrovascular disease Widely available in tertiary medical centers	In transfused HbSS subjects, velocities decrease to normal range Requires meticulous examination technique
Conventional MRI (cMRI)	Acute infarction visible on T1-weighted sequences as low attenuation, hyperintense T2 in completed and border zone incomplete infarction (silent infarction)	Widely available equipment allows high-resolution anatomic visualization of gray and white matter in cerebral infarction Requires modest technical experience	Confinement time in equipment is prolonged; use in unstable patients or during stroke in progression not recommended Poor identification of hemorrhage early
Diffusion- and perfusion-weighted MRI (MRI [DWI])	Identifies molecular displacement of water	Early hyperintense signal detection of acute ischemia before cMRI or CT is sensitive by 8 hours Identifies penumbral areas surrounding infarcts Can be incorporated into routine MRI procedure by adding 3 minutes to immobility time	Requires high-speed echoplanar imaging (EPI) with absolute immobility of head (single shot requires 100 ms)
Fluid-attenuated inversion recovery MRI (FLAIR)	Finer definition of neuronal microanatomy Special pulse sequence	Cerebrospinal fluid appears dark White matter lesions, acute infarcts appear bright	Axial sequence is required as a part of the routine brain protocol
Quantitative MRI (qMRI)	T1 (spin-lattice relaxation time) demonstrates subtle gray matter abnormalities in subjects with normal cMRI	Very high resolution using available equipment Good correlation with regional cognitive deficiencies	Requires special software and extensive radiologic expertise

Table 1: (continued)

Modality	Physiologic activity	Advantages	Disadvantages
MR spectroscopy (MRS)	Spectra measures brain lactate, glutamine, N-acetyl aspartate and other metabolites	Rapid onset but short lived elevation of lactate and glutamate with ischemia in gray matter before cMRI or CT abnormalities appear	Adult norms achieved by age 2 years Difficult clinical monitoring during critical period of stroke in progression Subject immobility required
MR angiography (MRA)	High-resolution visualization of stenotic carotid and intracerebral arteries	Good correlation to conventional angiography with less adverse risk Uses available MRI equipment with slight increase in time of confinement	Endothelial roughening and irregular blood flow velocity mimics stenosis
Computed tomography (CT)	Low-attenuation regions in completed infarctions Cerebral atrophy well defined	Short acquisition time Readily available Acute hemorrhage is hyperintense and identifiable within a few hours of onset	Incomplete (silent) border zone infarctions are often not identified

Data from Refs. [8,11,22,23,39–45,48].

Prevention

The ideal treatment for stroke is prevention [46]. Drugs such as hydroxyurea, decitabine, and apicidin [49] that increase the proportion of fetal hemoglobin (HbF) in the sickle red blood cell show promise. Hydroxyurea demonstrates a two-pronged effect by also decreasing HbS reticulocyte adhesion to the endothelium. There is solid theoretical support but no evidenced-based clinical trials to support its use in high-risk children to prevent cerebral ischemia [50].

Ideally, the fundamental requirement of successful management is treatment of the HbSS child before neuronal loss has begun. Bone marrow or stem cell transplantation is successful if engraftmentsucceeds. This highly invasive therapy is only possible in the 10% to 15% of children who have HLA-compatible siblings who are not HbSS.

Acute management

Immediate neuroprotective therapy includes control of oxygenation, blood pressure, dehydration, hypothermia, hyperglycemia, and aspiration. Cerebral ischemia and early reperfusion trigger a cascade of events that involve presynaptic release of glutamate, activation of proteases as a result of increased intracellular calcium, generation of free radicals, and subsequent inflammatory responses. Several neuroprotective agents, such as N-methyl D-aspartate receptor antagonists, glycine antagonists, calcium blockers and free radical scavengers, and anti-inflammatory agents, are under study in adult atherosclerotic patients [51,52]. Their function is to preserve the brain tissues in the penumbra areas during stroke in progression. None of these agents has been used in a research setting in patients with sickle cell anemia with infarctive stroke.

Transfusion therapy

The early onset of cerebral vasculopathy in HbSS children is directly related to the age-specific elevated cerebral blood flow and the increased oxygen required for brain maturation [53–55]. The magnitude of the damage is compounded by anemia, abnormal red blood cell rheology, and sickle reticulocyte-induced endothelial hyperplasia. If untreated, two of three children with clinical strokes will have repeat strokes [5]. The treatment of clinical stroke during childhood has generally relied on chronic transfusion therapy, often until the patient is at least 18 years of age. If maintained on HbA red blood cell transfusion, most patients sustaining hemiparetic hemisensory strokes will demonstrate fewer recurrent clinical episodes [21,56]. The goal of transfusion therapy is to maintain the hemoglobin concentration at 12 g/dL and the HbS percentage at less than 30%. In HbSS subjects with prior stroke, transfusion is associated with a 20% reduction in mean MCA blood flow velocities as measured by ultrasound [47]. These reductions occur rapidly within the first 3 hours of transfusion and are directly correlated with a rise in the hematocrit of 29% to 34%. Blood rheology immediately improves because of the dilution of sickle cells. Transfusion therapy should be initiated as soon as the diagnosis of cerebral infarction is confirmed. The choice as to the type of transfusion includes repeated simple transfusions of leukocyte-depleted cross-matched red cells, exchange transfusion, or erythrocytapheresis. Initially, simple transfusion is given during stroke in progression because of the fragile state of the child requiring intensive care monitoring. This transfusion can be followed by exchange transfusion, erythrocytapheresis, or repeat simple transfusion. The choice is usually based on institutional preference and resources. There are no outcome data to support any specific transfusion procedure.

The cerebral vasculopathy during the first decade is not a static process. On transfusion, some patients will show an improvement in functional neuroimaging during the first year of therapy, whereas others will develop new asymptomatic penumbral lesions [55,57]. MR angiography shows occasional smoothing of previously roughened endothelium in some transfused patients but progression of large vessel disease in others [58]. Completed infarction sites do not improve, and penumbral lesion progression occurs with continued loss of neuropsychologic function [9,24,31]. Functional neurologic deficits persist and become more obvious as the child matures. In children with elevated cerebral blood flow who are less than 10 years of age, stroke frequently recurs when the transfusion program is discontinued [3]. The consensus is that transfusion should continue until approximately 18 years of age or longer. Attempts to reduce the transfusion level after a number of years because of iron overload in older adolescents and young adults have been shown to be relatively safe. The hemoglobin S percentage is allowed to rise to approximately 50% [59].

Clearly, the prevention of first stroke should be a goal of therapeutic intervention [25,46]. Adams and coworkers initiated a randomized clinical trial directed at stroke prevention. Asymptomatic young children who had elevated blood flow velocity measured by transcranial Doppler imaging of the MCA or dICA (>200 cm/s) were randomized to receive transfusion or no transfusion. Within 2.5 years, the patients who were randomly assigned to transfusion therapy had fewer overt clinical strokes than those who were maintained on standard nontransfusion therapy (11 subjects with 10 cerebral infarctions and one intracranial hemorrhage in the nontransfusion group versus one cerebral infarction in the transfusion group), a 92% difference in stroke risk. The patients with concomitant abnormal conventional MRI were at highest risk for overt clinical infarction. In a second trial (STOP II), transfused subjects with no clinical evidence of a neurologic disorder but elevated Doppler velocity were randomized to discontinuance of transfusion therapy after 30 months. Sixteen of 41 patients randomized to discontinuance of transfusion therapy reverted to high-risk transcranial Doppler findings, and two subsequently had overt clinical strokes. The combination of increased MCA and dICA velocities along with evidence of persistence of the border zone MRI abnormalities mark a high rate of progressive neuropathy of 38%; therefore, transfusion therapy cannot be safely discontinued after 30 months [57]. Currently ongoing is a multi-institutional randomized study of red blood cell transfusions versus no transfusion in children identified by conventional MRI imaging to have asymptomatic incomplete infarctions without elevated Doppler velocities.

Chronic transfusion therapy is burdensome to the patient and family and is associated with a high frequency of problems [60]. Venous access becomes a major issue. Also added to the burden is increasing adolescent resistance to nightly subcutaneous chelation therapy, which is painful and difficult to continue over many years. Iron chelation therapy requires the use of subcutaneous or intravenous deferoxamine (Desferal). Complications include skin rash, ototoxity, and, in young children, growth retardation. Compliance with home treatment in adolescents is poor, limiting its usefulness. New (non–Food and Drug Administration approved) investigational agents include deferiprone alone or in combination with deferoxamine. Deferosirox, a tridentate iron chelator, is given orally at 20 mg/kg/day dissolved in water and has shown few toxicities in phase II studies to date with some nausea and vomiting. Effectiveness is assessed using superconducting quantum interference device (SQUID) measurements of liver iron. The parents need to be informed that embarkation on a transfusion program in this clinical situation is a long-term commitment, and compliance with an iron chelation regimen is vital.

Hydroxyurea

Hydroxyurea therapy may be useful as a replacement for transfusion [61,62]. The hematologic factors of elevated neutrophils, platelets, and reticulocyte count that predict an increased risk of cerebral vasculopathy also predict which subjects will respond best to hydroxyurea. The dose of hydroxyurea can be escalated from 15 to 35 mg/kg/day monitoring the hematologic parameters. The maximum dose for older children and adolescents is between 1000 and 1500 mg orally per day [63]. In HbSS adults without known stroke, hydroxyurea was shown to reduce the frequency of painful crisis, acute chest syndrome, and hospitalization, and the need for blood transfusion in a double-blind placebo-controlled study. Hydroxyurea decreased the risk of adult mortality in a 9-year follow-up study [64]. There are no controlled trials on the progression of cerebral vasculopathy during hydroxyurea therapy. Successful replacement of transfusion therapy with hydroxyurea in patients known to have symptomatic stroke who were unable to tolerate continued transfusion therapy has been reported [61,62,65,66]. It is thought that hydroxyurea may decrease the rate of penumbral spread to regions adjacent to already infarcted regions.

The question is whether hydroxyurea or similar agents can prevent the development of cerebral vasculopathy in the very young child. The fact that splenic germinal centers have been shown to return may be a promising model [67]. There are no data available regarding the efficacy of hydroxyurea therapy in the very young patient at 3 or 4 years in an attempt to prevent cerebral vasculopathy before clinical or radiologic evidence of central nervous system disease becomes apparent. Long-term clinical trials of hydroxyurea beginning during early childhood in a multi-institutional trial in North America are in progress [50]; however, recent neuroradiologic advances using conventional MRI or FLAIR imaging are not included in the trial. An evidenced-based randomized clinical trial monitored by neuroimaging and neuropsychologic testing is needed. To be clinically effective in the prevention of central nervous system vasculopathy, therapeutic agents must be relatively nontoxic in children, orally available, and should not impart an unpleasant odor (ie, butyrate). Long-term compliance with oral medication is a major difficulty in young children.

Published recommendations do not include data regarding seriously ill young adults with significant comorbid conditions such as renal insufficiency and chronic pulmonary disease who cannot be managed with the single focus on cerebral vasculopathy. Children who have had clinical stroke and who have been transfused for 10 to 15 years often have the complications of chronic transfusion, that is, iron overload with hemosiderosis of the liver and alloimmu-nization. They are frequently removed from the transfusion program, given hydroxyurea, and observed. No data are available on subjects regarding renal function or pulmonary function as their transfusion therapy is discontinued.

Neurorehabilitation

Rehabilitative techniques have advanced significantly during the last decade. Most large hospitals have neurorehabilitation services focusing on adult patients with stroke. These services have been underused by the pediatric population. The services go far beyond the standard physical therapy of muscle strengthening and treatment for poststroke spasticity and improvement of coordination and volitional movements [68,69]. Constraint-induced therapy has shown good success in the rehabilitation of adult patients [70]. It is possible to harness the plasticity of adaptive properties of neuronal networks in the brain through therapies that engage the patient in active voluntary use of impaired limbs [71]. Constraint-induced therapy is intended to help patients with central paresis overcome learned "nonuse" of the paretic limb and involves a physical restraint such as a mitt or sling on the functional arm or leg to encourage use of the nonfunctional extremity [70–72].

Studies are underway to determine whether the dopamine agonist ropinirole (Requip) combined with physical therapy can be associated with improved gait and motor status [73]. The hypothesis is that decreased dopamine has a role in poststroke motor deficits. If the dopamine can be increased, motor recovery is thought to be more likely. Numerous studies suggest that increasing noradrenergic activity after stroke improves motor outcome. Human trials of l-dopa and amphetamine have found significant treatment-related gains in motor status but have been marred by significant toxicities. Ropinirole or similar agents might provide the same neurobeneficial results with considerably less toxicity.

Once a patient has had an acute stroke, prevention of recurrence, close monitoring by means of imaging modalities, psychometric analyses, and ongoing rehabilitation with psychosocial support should be implemented. It is hoped that studies currently ongoing and those being planned will make significant inroads into the prevention, diagnosis, and management of HbSS individuals with cerebral infarction.

References

[1] Pegelow CH, Wang W, Granger S, et al. Silent infarcts in children with sickle cell anemia and abnormal cerebral artery velocity. Arch Neurol 2001;58:2017–21.

[2] Prengler M, Pavlakis SG, Prohovnik I, et al. Sickle cell disease: the neurological complications. Ann Neurol 2002;51:543–52.

[3] Grubb RL, Derdeyn CP, Fritsch SM, et al. Importance of hemodynamic factors in the prognosis of symptomatic carotid occlusion. JAMA 1998; 280:1055–60.

[4] Ohene-Frempong K, Weiner SJ, Sleeper LA, et al. the Cooperative Study of Sickle Cell Disease.

Cerebrovascular accidents in sickle cell disease: rates and risk factors. Blood 1998;91:228–94.

[5] Powars DR, Wilson B, Imbus C, et al. The natural history of stroke in sickle cell disease. Am J Med 1978;65:461–71.

[6] Adams RJ, Ohene-Frempong K. Wang W Sickle cell and the brain. Hematology (Am Soc Hematol Educ Program) 2001;31–46.

[7] Wang WC, Gallagher DM, Pegelow CH, et al. Multicenter comparison of magnetic resonance imaging and transcranial Doppler ultrasonography in the evaluation of the central nervous system in children with sickle cell disease. J Pediatr Hematol Oncol 2000;22:335–9.

[8] Steen RG, Emudianughe T, Hankins GM, et al. Brain imaging findings in pediatric patients with sickle cell disease. Radiology 2003;228: 216–25.

[9] Garcia JH, Lassen NJ, Weiller C, et al. Ischemic stroke and incomplete infarction. Stroke 1996; 27:761–5.

[10] Koshy M, Thomas C, Goodwin J. Vascular lesions in the central nervous system in sickle cell disease (neuropathology). JAAMP 1990;1:71–8.

[11] Powars DR, Conti PS, Wong WY, et al. Cerebral vasculopathy in sickle cell anemia: diagnostic contribution of positron emission tomography. Blood 1999;93:71–9.

[12] Driscoll MC, Hurlet A, Styles L, et al. Stroke risk in siblings with sickle cell anemia. Blood 2003; 101:2401–4.

[13] Hoppe C, Klitz W, Noble J, et al. Distinct HLA associations by stroke in children with sickle cell anemia. Blood 2003;101:2865–9.

[14] Hsu LL, Miller ST, Wright E, et al. Alpha thalassemia is associated with decreased risk of abnormal transcranial Doppler ultrasonography in children with sickle cell anemia. J Pediatr Hematol Oncol 2003;25:622–8.

[15] Huang W, Wang H, Kekuda R, et al. Transport of N-acetylaspartate by the Na+ dependent high-affinity dicarboxylate transporter NaDC3 and its relevance to the expression of the transporter in the brain. Pharmacology 2000;295: 392–403.

[16] Steen RG, Ogg RJ. Abnormally high levels of brain N-acetylaspartate in children with sickle cell disease. AJNR Am J Neuroradiol 2005;26: 463–8.

[17] Miller ST, Sleeper LA, Pegelow CH, et al. Prediction of adverse outcomes in children with sickle cell disease: a report from the Cooperative Study (CSSCD). N Engl J Med 2000;342:83–9.

[18] Glauser TA, Siegel MJ, Lee BCP, et al. Accuracy of neurologic examination and history in detecting evidence of MRI-diagnosed cerebral infarctions in children with sickle cell hemoglobinopathy. J Child Neurol 1995;10:88–92.

[19] Wang WC, Langston JW, Steen RG, et al. Abnormalities of the central nervous system in very young children with sickle cell anemia. J Pediatr 1998;132:994–8.

[20] Miller ST, Macklin EA, Pegelow CH, et al. Silent infarction as a risk factor for overt stroke in children with sickle cell anemia: a report from the Cooperative Study of Sickle Cell Disease. J Pediatr 2001;139:385–90.

[21] Scothorn DJ, Price C, Schwartz D, et al. Risk of recurrent stroke in children with sickle cell disease receiving blood transfusion therapy for at least five years after initial stroke. J Pediatr 2002;140:348–54.

[22] Kirkham FJ, Calamante F, Bynevelt M, et al. Perfusion magnetic resonance abnormalities in patients with sickle cell disease. Ann Neurol 2001; 49(4):477–85.

[23] Dobson SR, Holden KR, Nietert PJ, et al. Moyamoya syndrome in childhood sickle cell disease: a predictive factor for recurrent cerebrovascular events. Blood 2002;99:3144–50.

[24] Swift AV, Cohen MJ, Hynd GW, et al. Neuropsychologic impairment in children with sickle cell anemia. An Pediatr (Barc) 1989;84: 1077–85.

[25] Adams RJ. Stroke prevention and treatment in sickle cell disease. Arch Neurol 2001;58:565–8.

[26] Quinn CT, Rogers ZR, Buchanan GR. Survival of children with sickle cell disease. Blood 2004;103: 4023–7.

[27] Powars DR. Management of cerebral vasculopathy in children with sickle cell anaemia. Br J Haematol 2000;108:666–78.

[28] Earley CJ, Kittner SJ, Feeser BR, et al. Stroke in children and sickle-cell disease: Baltimore-Washington Cooperative Young Stroke Study. Neurology 1998;51:169–76.

[29] Gabis LV, Yangala R, Lenn NJ. Time lag to diagnosis of stroke in children. An Pediatr (Barc) 2002;110:924–8.

[30] Katz ML, Smith-Whitley K, Ruzek SB, et al. Knowledge of stroke risk, signs of stroke, and the need for stroke education among children with sickle cell disease and their caregivers. Ethn Health 2002;7:115–23.

[31] Armstrong FD, Thompson RJ Jr, Wang W, et al. Cognitive functioning and brain magnetic resonance imaging in children with sickle cell disease. An Pediatr (Barc) 1996; 97:864–70.

[32] Craft S, Schatz J, Glauser TA, et al. Neuropsychologic effects of stroke in children with sickle cell anemia. J Pediatr 1993;123:712–7.

[33] Bernaudin F, Verlhac S, Freard F, et al. Multicenter prospective study of children with sickle cell disease: radiographic and psychometric correlation. J Child Neurol 2000;15:333–43.

[34] Schatz J, White DA, Moinuddin A, et al. Lesion burden and cognitive morbidity in children with sickle cell disease. J Child Neurol 2002;17: 891–5.

[35] Pegelow CH, Macklin EA, Moser FG, et al. Longitudinal changes in brain magnetic resonance imaging findings in children with sickle cell disease. Blood 2002;99:3014–8.

[36] Adams RJ. Lessons from the stroke prevention trial in sickle cell anemia (STOP) study. J Child Neurol 2000;15:344–9.

[37] Abboud MR, Cure J, Granger S, et al. Magnetic resonance angiography in children with sickle cell disease and abnormal transcranial Doppler ultrasonography findings enrolled in the STOP study. Blood 2004;103:2822–6.

[38] Vermeer SE, Prins ND, den Heijer T, et al. Silent brain infarcts and the risk of dementia and cognitive decline. N Engl J Med 2003;348:1215–22.

[39] Moran CJ, Siegel MJ, DeBaun MR. Sickle cell disease: imaging of cerebrovascular complications. Radiology 1998;206:311–21.

[40] Mullins ME, Schaefer PW, Sorensen AG, et al. CT and conventional and diffusion-weighted MR imaging in acute stroke: study in 691 patients at presentation to the emergency department. Radiology 2002;224(2):356–60.

[41] Moritani T, Numaguchy Y, Lemer NB, et al. Sickle cell cerebrovascular disease: usual and unusual findings on MR imaging and MR angiography. Clin Imag 2004;28:173–86.

[42] Steen RG, Reddick WE, Mulhern RK, et al. Quantitative MRI of the brain in children with sickle cell disease reveals abnormalities unseen by conventional MRI. J Magn Reson Imaging 1998;8:535–43.

[43] Crisostomo RA, Garcia MM, Tong DC. Detection of diffusion-weighted MRI abnormalities in patients with transient ischemic attack: correlation with clinical characteristics. Stroke 2003;34:932–7.

[44] Schaefer PW, Ozsunar Y, He J, et al. Assessing tissue viability with MR diffusion and perfusion imaging. AJNR Am J Neuroradiol 2003;24(3):436–43.

[45] Kandeel AY, Zimmerman RA, Ohene-Frempong K. Comparison of magnetic resonance angiography and conventional angiography in sickle cell disease: clinical significance and reliability. Neuroradiology 1996;38:409–16.

[46] Adams RJ, Brambilla DJ, Granger S, et al. Stroke and conversion to high risk in children screened with transcranial Doppler ultrasound during the STOP study. Blood 2004;103:3689–94.

[47] Venketasubramanian N, Prohovnik I, Hurlet A, et al. Middle cerebral artery velocity changes during transfusion in sickle cell anemia. Stroke 1994;25:2153–8.

[48] Noguchi K, Ogawa T, Inugami A, et al. Acute subarachnoid hemorrhage: MR imaging with fluid-attenuated inversion recovery pulse sequences. Radiology 1995;196:773–7.

[49] Witt O, Monkemeyer S, Ronndahl G, et al. Induction of fetal hemoglobin expression by the histone-deacetylase inhibitor apicidin. Blood 2003;101:2001–7.

[50] Rogers ZR, Buchanan GR. Expanding the role of hydroxyurea in children with sickle cell disease. J Pediatr 2004;145:287–8.

[51] Brott T, Bogousslavsky J. Treatment of acute ischemic stroke. N Engl J Med 2000;343:710–22.

[52] Scheidtmann K, Fries W, Muller F, et al. Effect of levodopa in combination with physiotherapy on functional motor recovery after stroke: a prospective, randomized, double-blind study. Lancet 2001;358:787–90.

[53] Schoning M, Hartig B. Age dependence of total cerebral blood flow volume from childhood to adulthood. J Cereb Blood Flow Metab 1996;16:827–33.

[54] Huttenlocher PR, Moohr JW, Johns L, et al. Cerebral blood flow in sickle cerebrovascular disease. An Pediatr (Barc) 1984;73(5):615–21.

[55] Raj A, Bertolone SJ, Mangold S, et al. Assessment of cerebral tissue oxygenation in patients with sickle cell disease: effect of transfusion therapy. J Pediatr Hematol Oncol 2004;26:279–83.

[56] Buchanan GR, Bowman WP, Smith SJ. Recurrent cerebral ischemia during hypertransfusion therapy in sickle cell anemia. J Pediatr 1983;103:921–3.

[57] Pegelow CH, Adams RJ, McKie V, et al. Risk of recurrent stroke in patients with sickle cell disease treated with erythrocyte transfusions. J Pediatr 1995;126(6):896–9.

[58] Russell MO, Goldberg HI, Hodson A, et al. Effect of transfusion therapy on arteriographic abnormalities and on recurrence of stroke in sickle cell disease. Blood 1984;63(1):162–9.

[59] Cohen AR, Martin MB, Silber JH, et al. A modified transfusion program for prevention of stroke in sickle cell disease. Blood 1992;79:1657–61.

[60] Olivieri NF. Progression of iron overload in sickle cell disease. Semin Hematol 2001;38:57–62.

[61] Ware RE, Zimmerman SA, Schultz WH. Hydroxyurea as an alternative to blood transfusions for the prevention of recurrent stroke in children with sickle cell disease. Blood 1999;94:3022–6.

[62] Sumoza A, de Bisotti R, Sumoza D, et al. Hydroxyurea (HU) for prevention of recurrent stroke in sickle cell anemia (SCA). Am J Hematol 2002;71:161–5.

[63] Zimmerman SA, Schultz WH, Davis JS, et al. Sustained long-term hematologic efficacy of hydroxyurea at maximum tolerated dose in children with sickle cell disease. Blood 2004;103:2039–45.

[64] Steinberg MH, Barton F, Castro O, et al. Effect of hydroxyurea on mortality and morbidity in adult sickle cell anemia: risks and benefits up to 9 years of treatment. JAMA 2003;289:1645–51.

[65] Rana S, Houston PE, Surana N, et al. Discontinuation of long-term transfusion therapy in patients with sickle cell disease and stroke. J Pediatr 1997;131:757–60.

[66] Ware RE, Zimmerman SA, Sylvestre PB, et al. Prevention of secondary stroke and resolution of transfusional iron overload in children with

sickle cell anemia using hydroxyurea and phlebotomy. J Pediatr 2004;145:346–52.

[67] Wang WC, Wynn LW, Rogers ZR, et al. A two-year pilot trial of hydroxyurea in very young children with sickle-cell anemia. J Pediatr 2001;139: 790–6.

[68] Jackson PL, Lafleur MF, Malouin F, et al. Functional cerebral reorganization following motor sequence learning through mental practice with motor imagery. Neuroimage 2003;20: 1171–80.

[69] Stevens JA, Stoykov ME. Using motor imagery in the rehabilitation of hemiparesis. Arch Phys Med Rehabil 2003;84:1090–2.

[70] Taub E, Uswatte G, Pidikiti RD. Constraint-induced movement therapy: a new family of techniques with broad application to physical rehabilitation. A clinical review. J Rehab Res Dev 1999;36:237–51.

[71] Winstein CJ, Wing AM, Whitall J. Motor control and learning principles for rehabilitation of upper limb movements after brain injury. In: Grafman J, Robertson I, editors. Plasticity and rehabilitation. 2nd edition. (Handbook of neuropsychology, vol. 9). Amsterdam: Elsevier Science BV; 2003. p. 77–137.

[72] van der Lee J, Wagenaar R, Lankhorst G, et al. Forced use of the upper extremity in chronic stroke patients: results from a single-blind randomized clinical trial. Stroke 1999;30:2369–75.

[73] Gladstone DJ, Black SE. Enhancing recovery after stroke with noradrenergic pharmacotherapy: a new frontier? Can J Neurol Sci 2000;27: 97–105.

ELSEVIER
SAUNDERS

NEUROIMAGING
CLINICS
OF NORTH AMERICA

Neuroimag Clin N Am 17 (2007) 281–284

Index

Note: Page numbers of article titles are in **boldface** type.

1052-5149/07/$ – see front matter © 2007 Elsevier Inc. All rights reserved.
neuroimaging.theclinics.com

doi:10.1016/S1052-5149(07)00053-6

Moving?

Make sure your subscription moves with you!

To notify us of your new address, find your **Clinics Account Number** (located on your mailing label above your name), and contact customer service at:

E-mail: elspcs@elsevier.com

800-654-2452 (subscribers in the U.S. & Canada)
407-345-4000 (subscribers outside of the U.S. & Canada)

Fax number: 407-363-9661

Elsevier Periodicals Customer Service
6277 Sea Harbor Drive
Orlando, FL 32887-4800

*To ensure uninterrupted delivery of your subscription, please notify us at least 4 weeks in advance of move.